miracle foods

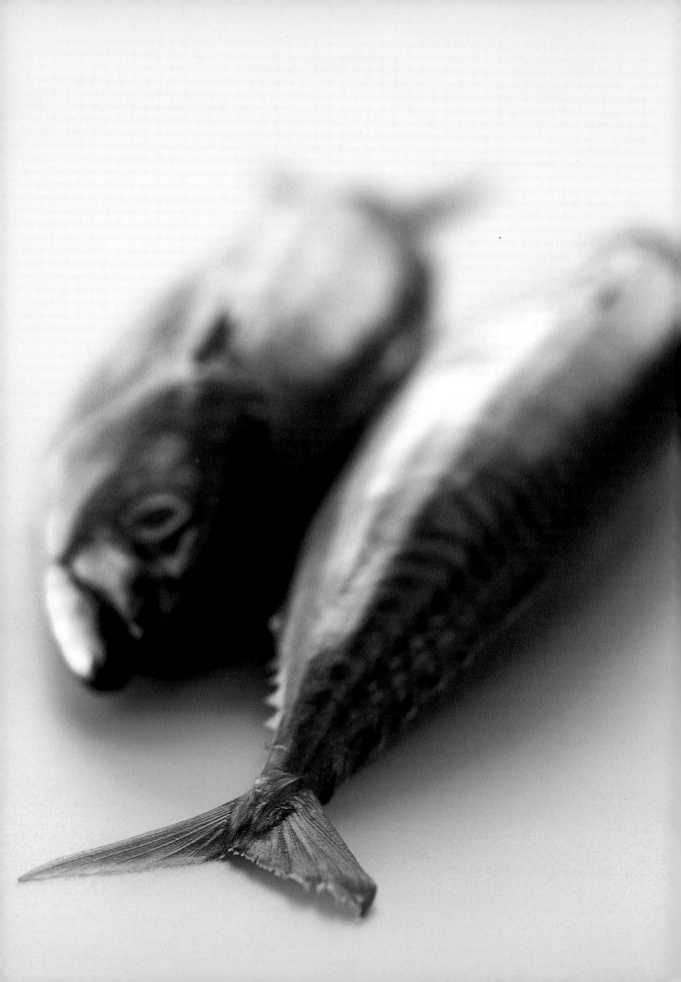

hamlyn

miracle foods

25 super-nutritious foods for great health!

Anna Selby

Recipes by Oona van den Berg

First published in 2001 by Hamlyn, an imprint
of Octopus Publishing Group Ltd
2-4 Heron Quays
London E14 4JP

ISBN 0 600 60192 7

A CIP catalogue record for this book is available from the British Library

Printed and bound in China

10 9 8 7 6 5 4 3 2 1

The publishers have taken all reasonable care in the preparation of this book but the
information it contains is not intended to take the place of treatment by a qualified medical
practitioner.

NOTES

1. Standard level spoon measurements are used in all recipes.
    1 tablespoon = one 15 ml spoon
    1 teaspoon = one 5 ml spoon
2. Imperial and metric measurements have been given in all recipes. Use one set of measurements only and not a mixture of both.
3. Measurements for canned food have been given as a standard metric equivalent.
4. Eggs should be large unless otherwise stated. The Department of Health advises that eggs should not be consumed raw. This book contains dishes made with raw or lightly cooked eggs. It is prudent for more vulnerable people, such as pregnant and nursing mothers, invalids, the elderly, babies and young children, to avoid dishes made with uncooked or lightly cooked eggs. Once prepared, these dishes should be kept refrigerated and used promptly.
5. Milk should be full-fat unless otherwise stated.
6. Fresh herbs should be used unless otherwise stated. If unavailable, use dried herbs as an alternative, but halve the quantities stated.
7. Pepper should be freshly ground black pepper unless otherwise stated.
8. Ovens should be preheated to the specified temperature – if using a fan-assisted oven, follow the manufacturer's instructions for adjusting the time and the temperature.
9. This book includes dishes made with nuts and nut derivatives. It is advisable for readers with known allergic reactions to nuts and nut derivatives and those who may be potentially vulnerable to these allergies, such as pregnant and nursing mothers, invalids, the elderly, babies and children, to avoid dishes made with nuts and nut oils. It is also prudent to check the labels of pre-prepared ingredients for the possible inclusion of nut derivatives.
10. Vegetarians should look for the 'V' symbol on a cheese to ensure that it is made with vegetarian rennet. There are vegetarian forms of Parmesan, feta, Cheddar, Cheshire, Red Leicester, dolcelatte and many goats' cheeses, among others.

contents

introduction

The food that we eat provides the raw materials and energy to power our extremely complex internal workings and the constant growth, repair and regeneration of our cells. Every day, our bodies are busy getting rid of old, damaged and dead cells and replacing them with new, healthy ones.

In order to keep our bodies healthy we should eat the foods that provide the best possible fuel and raw materials – 'Miracle Foods' – and avoid foods that might interfere with these processes or actively harm us.

WHY ARE SOME FOODS BAD FOR US?

Many of us eat processed or junk foods. Why are these so bad for us? As well as having little nutritional value, they contain too much fat, refined sugar and salt, and too many artificial colourings, flavourings and preservatives. We also drink coffee, tea and alcohol, and eat foods treated with systemic pesticides. Because of this our bodies react in the same way as they do when we are ill, concentrating on getting rid of the toxins and leaving less time and energy for the everyday processes of cleansing, healing and renewal. Over time the body can't keep up the pace. The strain shows first on the overworked liver, kidneys and immune system. The body's performance slows down and we become more susceptible to infection and ailments. We may end up overweight and unfit, with clogged-up arteries and heart disease, or cancer.

The World Health Organization has found that around 85 per cent of adult cancers are avoidable and, of these, around half are related to nutritional deficiencies in the Western diet.

The World Health Organization has said that vitamins A (beta-carotene from vegetable sources), C and E are vital for health.

These vitamins, together with the minerals selenium and zinc, are known as **antioxidants**. Many of the B-complex vitamins, enzymes and certain amino acids have antioxidant properties, too. They can protect us not only against minor infections, but also lower the risk of serious degenerative diseases, such as cancer and heart disease, as well as the conditions that come with premature ageing. They work by acting as scavengers for free radicals (see page 8).

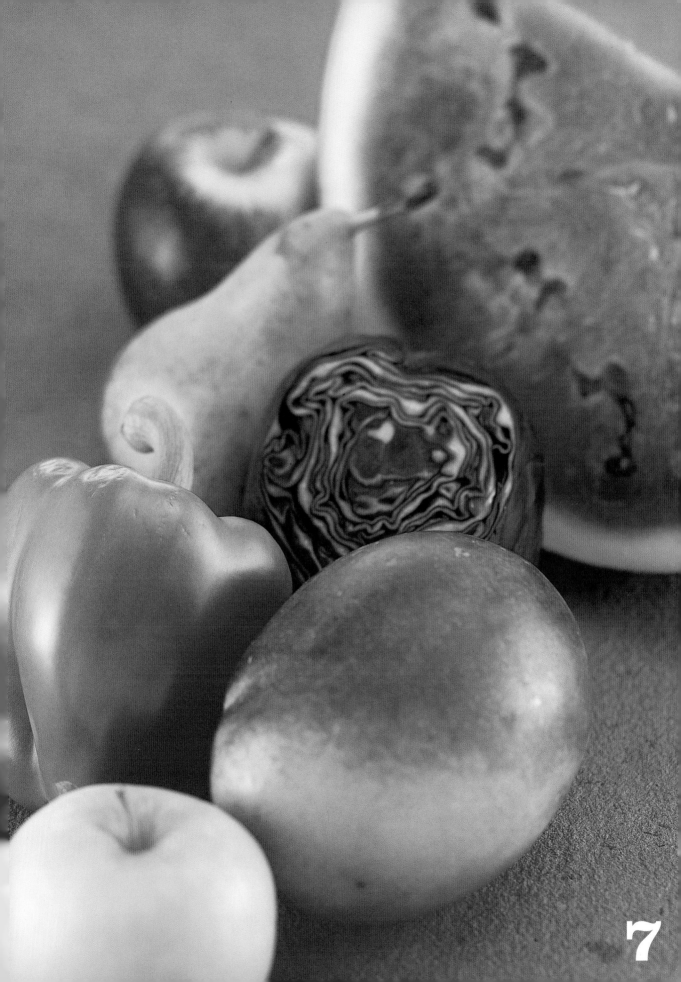

7

WHY ARE MIRACLE FOODS
SO GOOD FOR US?

Miracle Foods don't simply have a minimum of bad chemicals, but actually contain high amounts of beneficial substances that help to get rid of toxins and boost the immune system. Some of the most valuable of these foods are the subject of this book and in the following pages we look in more detail at just why they have such extraordinary powers to protect us from illness.

As well as being generally beneficial, the 25 foods and groups of foods featured have all been chosen because they are particularly valuable for combating particular health problems. For example,

nuts have high levels of vitamin E, which helps to protect against heart disease, and honey has such good antibacterial properties that the World Health Organization recommends it as a natural remedy for some gastric infections.

The recipes have been chosen because they include the various miracle foods and they use the healthiest cooking methods – steaming, stir-frying, baking and grilling. These cooking methods preserve the nutrients and health-giving properties, and bring out the full flavour of the food.

FOOD AND NUTRITION

It is important to choose good quality food, but it is equally important to eat a wide range of foods that combine to give your body the fuel it needs.

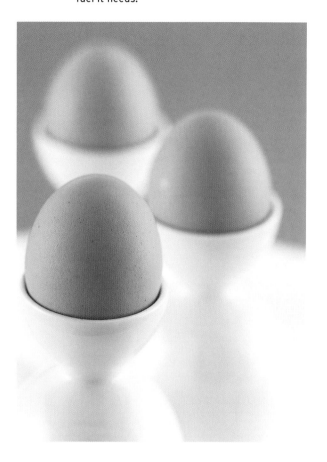

Protein

Proteins are found in fish, meat, poultry, game, dairy produce, eggs, beans and lentils, nuts, seeds and tofu. Proteins are vital for cellular growth and repair, but should form only about 10–15 per cent of the total diet. Some of these foods, such as red meat and eggs are also high in fat and so should be eaten in moderation. On the other hand, oily fish, such as salmon, mackerel, tuna and sardines, are extremely beneficial. Dairy produce can be eaten in moderation, but it is better to choose low-fat versions where available. Live yogurt is an excellent source of dairy protein as well as being generally beneficial to intestinal health.

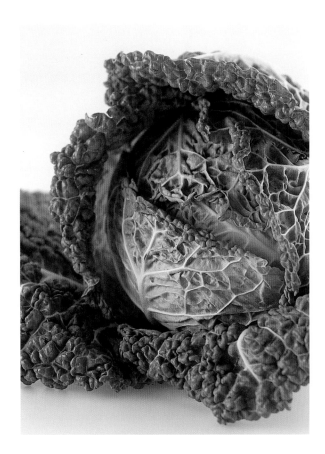

Starch

Starchy foods include cereals, such as wheat, rye, oats, barley and rice, and some vegetables, such as potatoes, sweet potatoes and yams. These complex carbohydrates should be the basis of your diet, making up about half of the food that you eat. People used to believe that these were the foods that made you overweight. In fact, depending on how they are prepared, they can help to control weight, as they satisfy hunger but are very low in fat. Eating a diet that is high in carbohydrates lowers the risk of having a stroke, heart disease, diabetes and several forms of cancer.

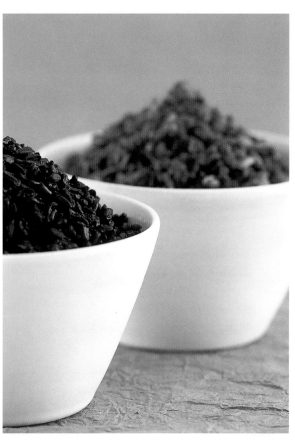

Fruit and vegetables

These contain many antioxidants (see page 6) (vitamins A, in beta-carotene form, C and E), as well as a range of minerals. They also form one of the best sources of fibre, as well as often having a high proportion of water – making them particularly beneficial in aiding digestion. You should include a wide range of fruit and vegetables in your diet.

Remember that the five portions of fruit and vegetables a day recommended by the World Health Organization should be treated as a minimum.

Red, yellow and orange fruits and vegetables, such as peppers, pineapples and carrots, have high levels of beta-carotene, from which our bodies produce vitamin A; while green, leafy vegetables, such as watercress, spinach and broccoli, are an excellent source, too, of vitamin C and and a whole range of minerals (see page 18).

Sugars

Sugar is a simple carbohydrate and nutritionally worthless. Foods or drinks with refined sugar can provide a quick burst of energy, it is true, but this would be better obtained in a natural form by eating a piece of fruit. Many sugary products, such as cakes, buns, sweet pastry and biscuits, are also high in fat. Sugar is much more pervasive than many of us realize. It is added as a preservative or flavouring to many prepared foods and drinks, including unlikely ones such as canned baked beans and processed peas.

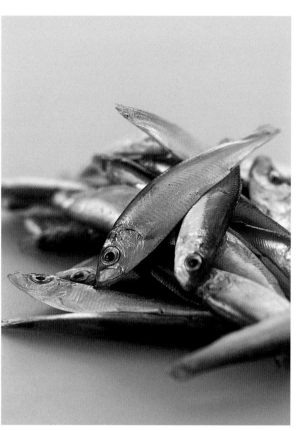

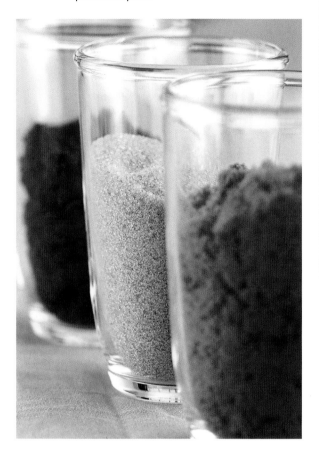

Fats

We do need some fat in our diet – it is the only source of essential fatty acids and it helps the absorption of vitamins A, D, E and K – but we only need a very small amount of the most beneficial types, such as olive and sesame oils.

There are three types of fat: saturated, monounsaturated and polyunsaturated. **Saturated fat** is the most dangerous kind, increasing the risk of a stroke, heart disease and also weight gain. It occurs in farmed meat and dairy produce, especially butter and hard cheeses.

Monounsaturated fats, such as olive oil, used in cooking are far more beneficial than the saturated fat alternatives. They support the beneficial high density lipoprotein (HDL) cholesterol in the blood.

Polyunsaturated fats are also known as the essential fatty acids. They reduce low density lipoprotein (LDL) cholesterol – the dangerous form of cholesterol – and are found most plentifully in oily fish, as well as some nuts and beans and a range of cooking oils, including safflower, sunflower and walnut.

Fibre

Everyone now knows that fibre is an essential element in our diets. However, this has led to many people having a high intake of bran-type cereals and, while these are certainly a form of fibre, they are not the best sort of fibre for the digestive system. They are often too abrasive, speeding up the digestive process unnaturally and inhibiting the absorption of several vital minerals and vitamins. The best form of fibre is in wholemeal bread, while probably the most obvious fibre is found in fruit and vegetables. They also contain many other useful vitamins and minerals, as well as a high proportion of water, which again is useful for digestion.

FOOD INTOLERANCE

There are also numerous foods, some of which seem highly beneficial, that cannot be tolerated by some individuals and interfere with their ability to absorb vital nutrients. This is known as a food intolerance and it is becoming an increasingly common problem. A food intolerance is not the same as a food allergy. Food allergies have a very sudden and dramatic effect, such as vomiting, a rash or, in severe cases, anaphylactic shock or even death.

Food intolerances, on the other hand, appear more slowly and have chronic, long-term symptoms. For this reason, they are sometimes referred to as hidden, masked or delayed allergies. The lengthy list of symptoms includes skin conditions, such as acne, eczema and psoriasis; digestive disorders, for example colitis and irritable bowel syndrome; weight problems; hyperactivity and other behavioural problems in children; rheumatoid arthritis and osteoarthritis; insomnia, headaches, migraine and exhaustion, and a range of psychological problems, such as depression.

One common culprit is wheat, and people whose diet centres on bread, cakes, biscuits and pasta can develop an intolerance to wheat. Processed foods, savoury snacks and sweets can also cause problems. Many of the foods which cause intolerances are, curiously, often staples in a person's diet or foods that they crave, such as chocolate or coffee. This is because the sufferer's body not only adapts to the intolerance, but becomes dependent on it. The food acts on the system as a toxin and the body, unable to absorb it in the normal way, reacts against it. Problems flare up elsewhere that seem quite unconnected with the offending food, especially as the reaction takes place several days later, so the culprit foods remain a mystery.

Further confusion is caused by the different effects that a food intolerance may have. Wheat, for instance, may cause migraine in one person, but eczema in another. Another problem is the multiplicity of symptoms. Typically, one person might have alternating constipation and diarrhoea, migraine, rheumatoid arthritis and a general feeling of such lassitude that he or she can hardly get out of bed in the morning.

One of the ways in which nutritionists pinpoint a food intolerance is by an elimination diet, in which a very bland diet is first established and then foods are introduced, one by one, to monitor whether they have an effect. If they don't, they can be included in the diet once more. If they do, this is clearly the sign of an intolerance and they should be excluded permanently.

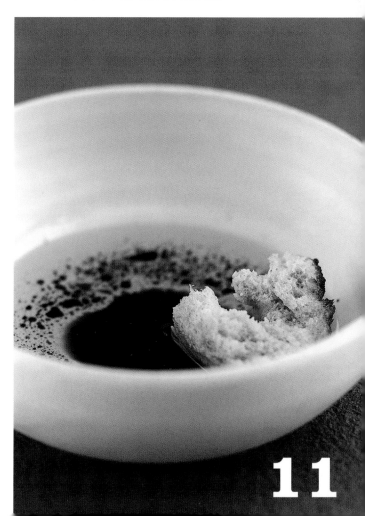

THE RIGHT FUEL

What is a good diet? There are a number of factors to consider here, but perhaps the most useful rule is to look for food that hasn't been processed in any way and is as close as possible to its natural state. This means avoiding the processed, ready-prepared foods that increasingly form the basis of the modern Western diet. So, instead of buying a piece of fish that has been covered in batter or breadcrumbs, look instead for a whole fresh fish, such as a trout or a mackerel, or a fillet from a larger fish, such as a salmon. Instead of refined flour, bread, pasta, rice and sugar, choose the whole, brown varieties. Ready-prepared meals, whether chilled or frozen, will often have a lot of additives to enhance their flavour and colour or extend their shelf life, and they may also be high in fat.

Pesticides and other chemicals

Even with unprocessed, fresh foods, is the hidden extras they might contain. Low levels of

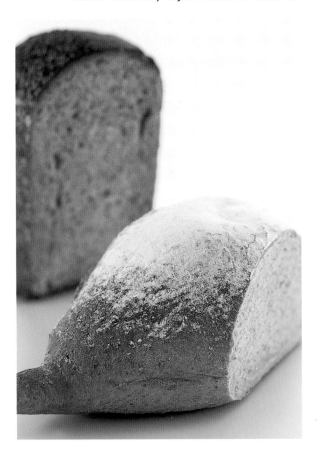

the chemicals used on foods are not likely to be actively harmful to the human system. However, it seems unlikely that they are beneficial and the question of whether organic food is better for you has become a controversial issue in some parts of the world and will doubtless remain so for some time. If you are worried about the idea of eating food that may contain chemicals, try to buy organic foods whenever possible.

Fresh food

The fresher your food is, the better it is for you, because all foods lose nutrients over time. Ideally, fish and shellfish should be eaten the day you buy them or the following one; poultry and lean meat can be kept for two days. These foods can be frozen, as they do not lose much nutritional value, but do this the day you buy them. Always make sure frozen food is adequately thawed before you cook it and always cook fish and meat thoroughly. Fruit and vegetables should be bought regularly and used as soon as possible.

If organic crops are available, do buy them. Modern systemic pesticides and fungicides work their way into the whole plant, rather than remaining on the surface and so can't be removed by washing.

Storing foods

Dried foods, such as pulses and seeds, should be eaten within six months, and preferably more quickly. Oils should be stored in dark glass rather than clear glass and kept in a dark cupboard to prevent oxidation. Olive oil lasts better than most, but all oils should be used in a matter of weeks rather than months. As a rule it is better to use glass containers rather than plastic, as foods may absorb chemicals from the latter.

Whole foods

Because there are many vital vitamins and minerals just beneath the surface of the skin, whenever possible, fruit and vegetables should

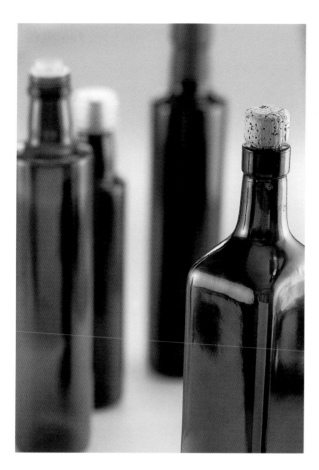

Boiling

Overcooked vegetables are not only soggy and tasteless, they have also been deprived of most of their vitamins and minerals. When boiling them use as little water as possible, boil the water before adding the vegetables and cook them for as short a time as possible. Most green vegetables will be ready for eating after just a few minutes' boiling. Don't add salt to the cooking water, as this not only adds more salt to your diet but leaches nutrients from the vegetables by drawing water from them, and always use a lid to stop steam escaping. Don't throw away the water – it is useful for making stocks, sauces and gravy.

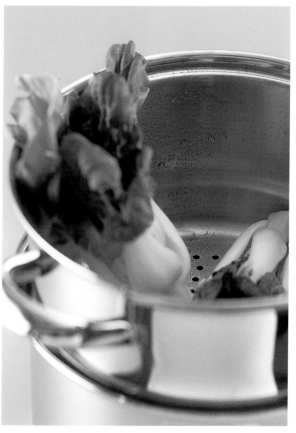

be eaten whole, rather than peeled. Potatoes, carrots and sweet potatoes don't usually need more than a good scrub to remove dirt or residual chemicals, although some foods with very tough skins – such as yams – will need have their skin removed before cooking. Never soak fruit or vegetables, as they will lose nutrients in the water.

PREPARING AND EATING FOOD

Chop fruit or vegetables just before you cook them or make them into a salad. Once they have been chopped up, they are subject to oxidation, which destroys their nutrients. Similarly, cooked meals should be eaten straightaway rather than left and reheated later. How you prepare and eat your food is important too. Many nutrients are needlessly lost during the cooking process, so raw food and raw juices (see page 16) are considered to be the most nutritionally beneficial for you.

Steaming

Steaming is an even better method of cooking vegetables. It takes only slightly longer and prevents the food's nutrients leaching into the water. Even dense root vegetables, such as potatoes, carrots, parsnips and sweet potatoes, can be steamed successfully.

Other Cooking Methods

Baking is a good method for retaining optimum nutrition. Stir-frying is another good option because the cooking process is so quick and usually requires only a little oil. If you want to use oil, then olive oil is best for cooking at high temperatures.

APPETIZERS

For people with small appetites, especially the elderly or convalescents, it is a good idea to try stimulating the digestive juices to encourage them to want to eat. A small green salad as a first course can do this – include salad vegetables such as rocket, watercress, parsley and other herbs.

WATER

While you can't classify water strictly as a food, it is essential to life. Water is needed for the smooth functioning of the body. Without enough water, body and mind become sluggish and less efficient.

How much water?

Our bodies are – or should be – at least 70 per cent water. However, because we lose water all the time, through urination, every time we breathe out and a staggering 1 litre (1¾ pints) per day through the skin alone.

We need to drink a minimum of 2 litres (3½ pints, or about 8 glasses) of water during a day, to keep our water level constantly replenished.

You will need even more if:
- the weather is very hot
- if you work in a centrally-heated or air-conditioned environment
- when you exercise
- when you travel by air

Unfortunately, many people don't drink enough water because they believe that drinking any fluid will do. Nothing could be further from the truth. Some popular drinks, such as coffee, actually dehydrate the body.

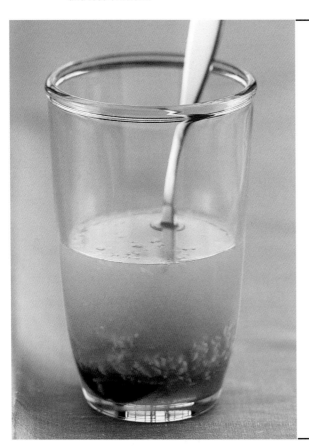

ginger pickle

An Ayurvedic (traditional Indian healthcare) way to stimulate the digestive juices is to eat a teaspoonful of ginger pickle 15 minutes before a meal. This recipe will make enough ginger pickle for several aperitifs and you can store it in the refrigerator. Always stir it again before taking your teaspoonful.

1 cm (½ inch) piece of fresh root ginger
4 tablespoons lemon juice
1 tablespoon clear organic honey
salt

1 Finely chop the ginger, put it into small bowl and pour the lemon juice over. Stir in the honey and a pinch of salt. If you do not find it sweet enough, add more honey.

While an occasional cup of tea or coffee or glass of wine is not going to harm you, the only liquid that is really going to hydrate you is water itself. Another good reason for avoiding alcoholic drinks and coffee is that they reduce the ability of the body to absorb vitamins. Tea blocks the absorption of iron, so should never be drunk with meals as the iron intake from the food will be greatly reduced.

Bottled water

If you drink bottled water, always make sure it states on the label that it's mineral water and that it contains beneficial minerals - in particular magnesium and calcium. Bottled waters called 'table waters' are not necessarily mineral waters at all.

Hard and soft water

People who live in hard water areas are 10-15 per cent less likely to suffer heart attacks or strokes than those who live in soft water areas, where the water supply does not contain the important minerals, and is more likely to absorb harmful metals from water pipes.

Water filters and softeners

You could invest in a good water filter - one that connects to the supply under the kitchen sink. This supplies pure water for cooking and drinking - particularly important if you are boiling vegetables or making soups or stews. Check that it takes out undesirable contaminants but leaves vital minerals in

CAFFEINE AND ALCOHOL

Coffee is a very effective diuretic, increasing urination levels, so the more you drink, the more fluids you lose. It also robs the body of precious minerals, such as magnesium, and blocks the body's ability to absorb vitamins. Caffeine does not only occur in coffee, it's in tea and cola drinks, too. Alcohol is another well-known dehydrator - just think of the raging thirst that accompanies a hangover.

place. If you use a chemical water softener to prevent limescale building up in your appliances, do not use this water for drinking or cooking.

BENEFICIAL TEAS

There are various ways of making water more interesting without adding to it damaging substances, such as caffeine. The best way is by

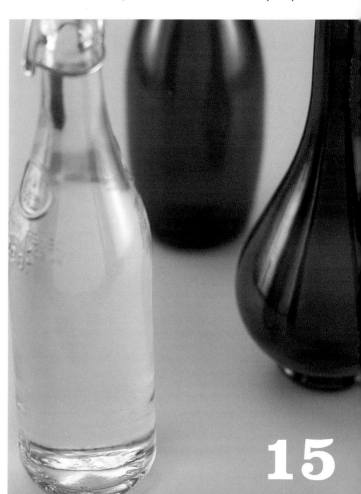

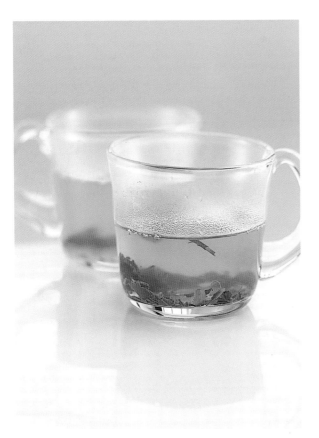

RAW JUICES

One of the best ways to make use of the nutrients in fruit and vegetables is to make your own fresh juices. It is, after all, a lot easier to drink a glass of carrot juice than munch your way through a bag of carrots! In addition, the body absorbs nutrients from liquid foods more rapidly and efficiently than if they are taken in the form of mineral and vitamin supplements.

Juices can be made from almost any fruit or vegetable imaginable, giving you a power-packed nutritional drink with a wide range of health-protecting properties.

To make them, you really need a juicing machine - food processors and blenders don't do the job as well unless you have a juicing attachment.

Protection against disease

The antioxidant vitamins found in fruit and vegetables protect the body not only against minor infections, but also against more serious conditions, including cancer and heart disease. The only thing that is lost in the juicing process is fibre and for this reason it is important to eat fruit and vegetables, as well as drink their juice.

What to juice?

You can juice almost all fruits and vegetables, but ensure that you mix them well so that you end up with a palatable taste. Many vegetables - particularly green vegetables - have very strong or bitter flavours and so only a small amount of these should be mixed with sweeter flavours, such as carrot or beetroot.

Look for fresh, seasonal fruits and vegetables. You can experiment simply by choosing your favourites and gradually bringing in other flavours to mix with them. Consider combinations used in salads as a guide to balancing flavours.

drinking herbal teas, such as peppermint or chamomile, or those made from fruits or spices. The ingredients in the tea are often beneficial in themselves. Peppermint, for instance, is good for the digestion and particularly helpful in quelling nausea. Chamomile improves sleep, while ginger benefits respiratory ailments and is a general stimulant.

Green tea comes from the same plant as ordinary black tea, but its leaves are pan-fried or steamed rather than fermented, as with black tea. It contains much less caffeine, and it does have vitamins, minerals and some powerful antioxidants called polyphenols. These are free-radical scavengers (see page 8) and can lower blood pressure, thus reducing the risk of a stroke and heart disease. Claims have been made, too, that green tea reduces the risk of lung, colon and stomach cancers, as well as breaking down fat and so helping with weight loss.

Top fruits and vegetables for juicing

Apples, carrots, strawberries, beetroot, pears, spinach, melon, peppers, pineapple and tomato – see below for a healthy juice using pineapples.

How to juice

A juicer divides the juices from the tougher pulp, pouring them into a cup. The juice should be drunk immediately, as it begins to oxidize and lose nutrients as soon as it has been made.

Use the whole fruit or vegetable. With the exception of very large and hard stones, seeds and pips should be juiced, too. Skins and rind, unless they are very tough, can also be juiced. Leaves on vegetables such as carrots, beetroot or celery often contain extra nutrients, so they should be included.

orange, banana and pineapple juice

Packed with vitamins A and C, magnesium, potassium and fibre, this juice will set you up for the day. You could also add a teaspoon of spirulina powder, a blue-green algae, for added bonus.

Preparation time: 5 minutes
Serves 2–4

2 oranges
150 g (5 oz) fresh pineapple or
**   1 queen pineapple**
2 bananas
450 ml (¾ pint) apple juice

1 Cut the rind and pith off the oranges and roughly chop the flesh.

2 Cut off the skin and cut out the eyes of the pineapple. Chop the flesh and put it into a juicer with the oranges, then process.

3 Transfer the juice to a food processor or blender. Peel the bananas, roughly chop the flesh and add to the food processor with the apple juice. Blend for 1 minute until smooth. Serve immediately.

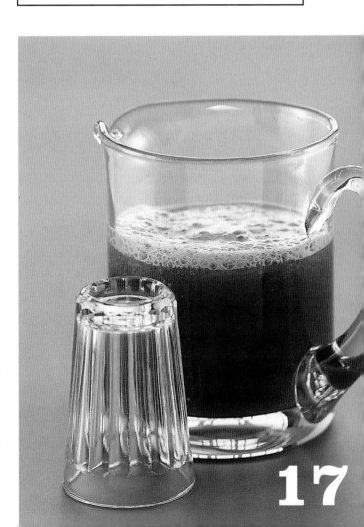

vitamins & minerals

Vitamin A (Retinol) Apples & Pears, Bananas, Beetroot, Berries, Broccoli, Cabbage, Carrots, Cashews, Chestnuts, Hazelnuts, Oily fish, Papayas, Peppers, Spinach, Sunflower seeds, Sweet potatoes, Tomatoes, Watercress

Vitamin B1 (Thiamine) Brazil nuts, Game, Oatmeal, Peanuts, Soya, Wholemeal bread

Vitamin B2 (Riboflavin) Almonds, Broccoli, Cheese, Game, Milk

Vitamin B3 (Niacin) Game, Mushrooms, Oily fish, Peanuts, Soya, Wholemeal bread

Vitamin B5 Broccoli, Game

Vitamin B6 (Pyridoxine) Bananas, Beetroot, Game, Hazelnuts, Soya

Vitamin B12 Cheese, Eggs, Game, Yeast extract

Vitamin C (Ascorbic acid) Apples & Pears, Bananas, Beetroot, Berries, Brazil nuts, Broccoli, Cabbage, Carrots, Chestnuts, Coconuts, Garlic, Hazelnuts, Honey, Leafy green vegetables, Mangoes, Papayas, Peppers, Spinach, Sweet potatoes, Tomatoes, Watercress

Vitamin D Cheese, Egg yolk, Milk, Oily fish, Sunflower seeds

Vitamin E Berries, Cabbage, Nuts, Mangoes, Olive oil, Papayas, Peppers, Sunflower and Sesame seeds, Spinach, Sweet potatoes, Tomatoes, Watercress

Vitamin K Spinach, Sunflower seeds

Folic acid Apples & Pears, Beans & Lentils, Beetroot, Broccoli, Coconuts, Sesame seeds, Spinach, Sweet potatoes, Watercress

Calcium Almonds, Apples & Pears, Beans & Lentils, Beetroot, Berries, Cabbage, Carrots, Cashews, Oats, Pumpkin and Sesame seeds, Seaweed & Sea vegetables, Soya & Tofu, Spinach, Sweet potatoes, Sunflower, Walnuts, Watercress, Yogurt

Copper Seaweed & Sea vegetables

Iodine Pears, Seaweed & Sea vegetables, Watercress

Iron Beans & Lentils, Beetroot, Berries, Broccoli, Game, Mangoes, Papayas, Pumpkin and Sesame seeds, Seaweed & Sea vegetables, Soya, Sunflower, Sweet potatoes, Watercress

Manganese Beans & Lentils, Beetroot, Spinach

Magnesium Apples & Pears, Beans & Lentils, Beetroot, Berries, Cabbage, Peppers, Pumpkin and Sesame seeds, Seaweed & Sea vegetables, Soya, Spinach, Sweet potatoes

Potassium Apples & Pears, Beans & Lentils, Beetroot, Berries, Seaweed & Sea vegetables, Soya, Spinach, Sweet potatoes

Phosphorus Apples & Pears, Beetroot, Oats, Soya & Tofu, Sweet potatoes

Selenium Beans & Lentils, Brazil nuts, Game, Oily fish, Sesame seeds, Soya, Walnuts

Silicon Seaweed & Sea vegetables

Zinc Almonds, Berries, Broccoli, Game, Hazelnuts, Mangoes, Papayas, Pine nuts, Pumpkin and Sesame seeds, Seaweed & Sea vegetables, Sunflower, Soya & Tofu, Sweet potatoes, Tomatoes, Watercress

foods for health

If you suffer from any of the complaints or conditions in this chart, it is recommended that you eat more of the suggested foods.

Anxiety & depression Bananas, Broccoli, Oats

Cancer (These foods help protect against the risk of cancer.) Bananas, Beans & Lentils, Broccoli, Cabbage, Oats, Oily fish, Olive oil, Papayas & Mangoes, Peppers, Seeds, Soya & Tofu, Spinach, Sweet potatoes, Tomatoes, Watercress

Cholesterol (To reduce) Apples, Bananas, Beans & Lentils, Garlic, Nuts, Oats, Oily fish, Olive oil, Soya & Tofu, Watercress, Yogurt

Circulatory problems & anaemia Beetroot, Blackberries, Blackcurrants, Blueberries, Redcurrants, Cabbage, Carrots, Game, Garlic, Honey, Nuts, Oats, Papayas & Mangoes, Spinach, Sweet potatoes, Tomatoes, Watercress

Detoxifying (These foods help prevent build-up of toxins.) Apples & Pears, Beans & Lentils, Broccoli, Carrots, Spinach, Sweet potatoes, Watercress

Digestive problems Apples & Pears, Bananas, Beans & Lentils, Broccoli, Cabbage, Carrots, Garlic, Honey, Linseeds, Oats, Olive oil, Papayas & Mangoes, Raspberries, Seeds, Soya & Tofu, Spinach, Sweet potatoes, Tomatoes, Watercress, Yogurt

Energy deficiency Apples & Pears, Bananas, Blackberries, Broccoli, Honey, Nuts, Papayas & Mangoes, Peppers, Spinach, Sweet potatoes & Yams, Watercress

Eyesight Carrots, Spinach, Sunflower seeds

Heart disease and stroke/high blood pressure (These foods lower the risk of heart disease and stroke and help reduce high blood pressure.) Bananas, Broccoli, Carrots, Garlic, Nuts, Oily fish, Olive oil, Peppers, Seaweed & Sea vegetables, Seeds, Soya & Tofu, Spinach, Sweet potatoes, Tomatoes, Watercress

Immune system deficiency Apples & Pears, Beetroot, Broccoli, Cabbage, Carrots, Game, Garlic, Honey, Oily fish, Papayas & Mangoes, Peppers, Seaweed & Sea vegetables, Seeds, Spinach, Sweet potatoes, Tomatoes, Watercress

Kidney, liver, bladder & urinary infections Beans & Lentils, Beetroot, Blackcurrants, Broccoli, Cabbage, Carrots, Chickpeas, Cranberries, Garlic, Honey, Sweet potatoes, Tomatoes, Watercress, Yogurt

PMS/Menstrual problems Bananas, Beans & Lentils, Beetroot, Berries, Carrots, Linseeds, Soya & Tofu, Yams, Nuts, Oats, Oily fish

Nervous system Bananas, Broccoli, Cabbage, Game, Nuts, Oats, Seaweed & Sea vegetables, Seeds, Spinach, Sweet potatoes, Watercress

Prostate problems Pumpkin seeds, Tomatoes

Respiratory problems/coughs & colds Apples, Blackberries, Broccoli, Cabbage, Carrots, Cranberries, Garlic, Honey, Olive oil

Rheumatism & rheumatoid arthritis Apples, Beans & Lentils, Honey, Nuts, Oily fish, Seeds, Strawberries

Skin conditions Apples & Pears, Broccoli, Cabbage, Carrots, Nuts, Oily fish, Olive oil, Papayas & Mangoes, Strawberries (see Berries), Sweet potatoes, Watercress

Sleeping problems Bananas

Strong teeth, bones, connective tissue (These foods help to build strong teeth, bones etc.) Carrots, Oats, Oily fish, Papayas & Mangoes, Soya & Tofu, Spinach, Sweet potatoes, Watercress

Thyroid problems Cabbage, Oats, Pears, Seaweed & Sea vegetables, Watercress

miracle food

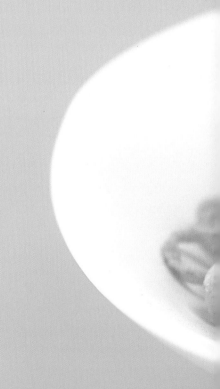

s & recipes

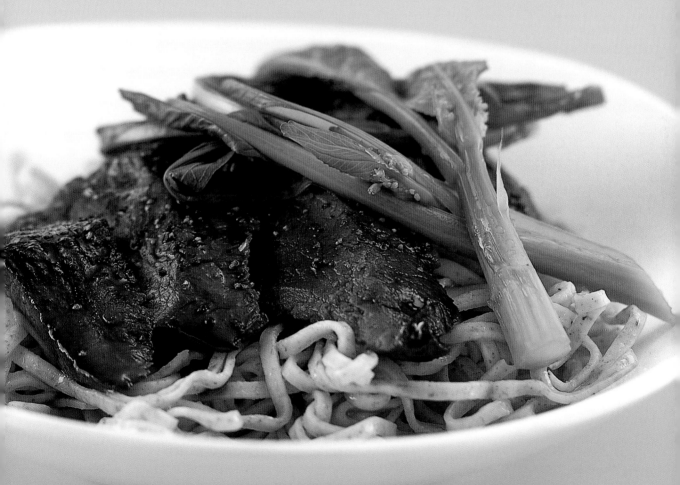

apples & pears

These are such common fruits that they often get taken for granted in the search for new and exotic tastes. In fact, they are packed with important vitamins and minerals and have valuable antioxidant effects.

Deep cleansing

One of the great advantages of both of these fruits is that they are profoundly detoxifying, in particular for the digestive system. In fact, you can give your whole body a programme of deep cleansing simply by eating nothing but apples and pears for a day. Both fruits are of benefit to your skin; whether you eat them whole and raw or drink them as juice, they will give you a healthy glow.

Besides ridding the body of toxins, apples and pears also strengthen the immune system helping it to resist infection. Pears are particularly cleansing and have a high iodine content which can aid thyroid function. Apples reduce cholesterol and also various forms of inflammation, most notably rheumatism, as well as soothing any inflammation caused by respiratory infection.

A healthy colon

Both apples and pears contain pectin, a soluble fibre that encourages peristalsis – the muscular contractions of the bowel – and this, in turn, helps to keep the colon healthy. Both fruits are gently laxative and diuretic. Apples contain enzymes that aid the digestive process and are believed by many naturopathic practitioners to help sufferers from irritable bowel syndrome (IBS) by relieving many of the symptoms that cause such discomfort. The fibre contained in fruits and vegetables is, in fact, increasingly regarded as more beneficial for the digestive system are the 'high fibre' cereals on sale in supermarkets, which can be far too harsh on the intestinal tract for people prone to digestive upsets. Both for their colon cleansing qualities and their energizing effects, apples and pears make an excellent start to the day. Include them either as part of your regular breakfast or, for those on a weight-loss diet, chopped into a fruit salad with some with low-fat yogurt and a scattering of seeds on top.

Choosing and storing

Buy organic fruit whenever possible. It may not be so blemish-free as the sprayed crops, but you know there will be no residual insecticides or pesticides. Buy fruit that is ripe. Many supermarkets sell fruit that has been picked too early and, while this prolongs its shelf life, fruit that is picked before it is ripe will not have developed its optimum nutritional value. Look for unbruised, firm-skinned fruits, avoiding any that look wrinkled or dried out, and always wash them thoroughly before eating. Although this has no effect on pesticides, it does remove dirt and germs acquired in handling.

There are both dessert and cooking varieties. Eat the dessert varieties raw with the skin on for maximum nutritional benefits and, if you make them into juice, use raw, whole fruit, including the pips. Avoid keeping fruit too long after purchase – the fresher it is when you eat it, the better – and try to keep it cool and out of direct sunlight, refrigerating it in hot weather.

The Benefits
- **Reduce cholesterol**
- **Cleanse the digestive system**
- **Provide many vitamins and minerals, notably beta-carotene, vitamin C, folic acid, calcium, magnesium, iodine, phosphorus, potassium**
- **Stimulate thyroid function (pears)**
- **Boost immune system**
- **Reduce inflammation**
- **Improve energy levels**

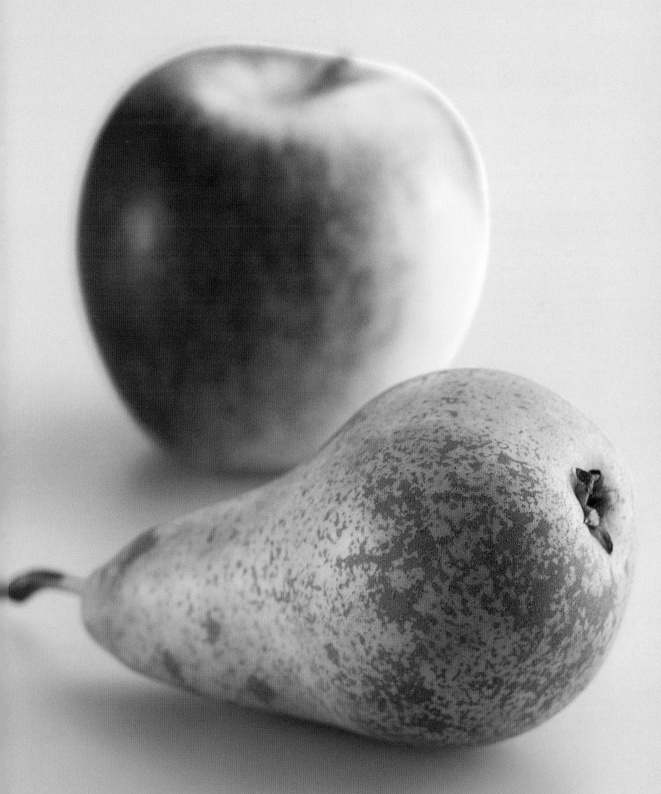

apple & hazelnut peasant girl in a veil

This is a very simple, old-fashioned pudding. The apple purée is sweetened with honey and has a hint of lemon from the rind added during cooking. The breadcrumbs, which can be white if you prefer, are better if the bread is a day or so old and slightly dry. Do not chill the pudding for too long or the breadcrumb layers will become soggy.

Preparation time: 20 minutes, plus chilling (optional)
Cooking time: 30 minutes
Serves 6

3 cooking apples
5 cm (2 inch) piece of lemon rind
1 tablespoon apple juice or water
1½ teaspoons grated fresh root ginger
50 g (2 oz) sultanas
1–2 tablespoons clear honey
75 g (3 oz) wholemeal breadcrumbs
2 tablespoons soft light brown sugar
50 g (2 oz) toasted hazelnuts, finely chopped
1 teaspoon ground cinnamon, to decorate
crème fraîche, yogurt or fromage frais, to serve (optional)

1 Peel the apples, core and roughly chop the flesh. Place it in a saucepan with the lemon rind, apple juice or water and ginger, and heat gently until the apple pieces begin to soften, stirring occasionally.

2 Once the juices have begun to ooze from the apples, add the sultanas, cover the pan with a lid and simmer gently for 10–15 minutes or until the apple has cooked through and become light and fluffy. Remove from the heat and beat with a wooden spoon to make a slightly coarse purée. Add honey to taste and remove and discard the lemon rind.

3 Heat a large frying pan until hot, add the breadcrumbs and toast, stirring constantly, until they are a light golden colour. Add the sugar and chopped hazelnuts, then remove the pan from the heat, still stirring constantly. Set aside to cool.

4 When the breadcrumb and nut mixture has cooled, break it into crumbs with the back of a spoon. Spoon 2 tablespoons of the apple purée into each of 4 small glasses, then cover with a layer of the breadcrumb and nut mixture. Repeat with the remaining apple and breadcrumb mixture.

5 Either serve immediately or chill for 1 hour. Just before eating, dust the puddings with the ground cinnamon and serve with crème fraîche, yogurt or fromage frais, if you like.

pear & parma ham open sandwiches with honey mustard

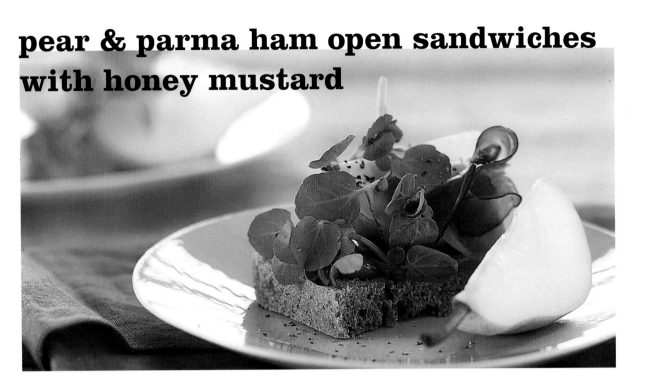

These substantial open sandwiches should be made and then eaten straightaway to prevent the pears from turning brown and the watercress from wilting. Fresh and packed with flavour, they make an ideal lunch or light supper.

Preparation time: 15 minutes
Serves 2

3 tablespoons thick honey
1 tablespoon Dijon mustard
2 teaspoons soft dark
    brown sugar
4 thick slices of Russian or
    German sourdough rye bread
1 ripe but firm Conference or
    Williams pear
4 slices Parma ham
large handful of watercress
pepper

1 Mix together the honey, mustard and soft brown sugar to make a smooth paste.

2 Spread the honey mustard over the slices of bread. Cut the pear in half lengthways without peeling it, core it and discard the pips, then cut it into thick slices.

3 Cover each piece of bread with slices of pear and then the slices of Parma ham. Add a pile of watercress leaves and grind pepper over the top. Serve straightaway with knives and forks.

bananas

Besides being delicious to eat, bananas are powerhouses of nutrition and energy. They make an ideal snack during the day if your energy starts to flag and they often satisfy a sweet craving in a healthy way.

Energy source

Bananas are an unusually rich fruit source of protein, and their energizing qualities make them a good fruit to breakfast or snack on. Compared to other fruits, they are rather high in calories (100 g/3½ oz of banana have 79 calories, compared to 46 for apples or 41 for pears) and fibre content, making them mildly laxative. Paradoxically, besides being energizing, bananas contain tryptophan, an amino acid with naturally sedative effects, which makes them a good bedtime snack for anyone who has trouble sleeping. Tryptophan is also a natural mood enhancer and raising tryptophan levels may alleviate symptoms of depression, anxiety and PMS.

Positive benefits

As well as their energizing-sedative benefits, bananas seem to have all-round beneficial effects on the body, depending on its needs. Their high potassium content, for instance, helps cellular growth and helps in controlling blood pressure, the smooth functioning of the nervous system and in regulating bodily fluids and the acid-alkali balance in the body.

Bananas also score high on vital antioxidants, notably beta-carotene, which converts naturally within the body to vitamin A, and vitamin C. Both of these vitamins offer protection against infection, as they boost the immune system, and also against heart disease and certain cancers. Bananas contain vitamin B6 too, another protector against heart disease, which regulates the nervous system and may help alleviate menstrual and menopausal problems as it helps produce the amino acids that control mood (see tryptophan above). Very ripe bananas are good for easing the symptoms of diarrhoea.

A gentle food

Bananas' all-round benefits and the fact that for most people they are an easily digested food make them an ideal 'starter food' for babies, so they are often given as one of the first solid foods, well mashed up with milk. Foods other than milk can be offered when babies reach 4-6 months, unless there are allergies in the family, where it would be advised to wait until 6 months in case a food intolerance occurs. As a general tonic, bananas are a good convalescence food and beneficial for people with low appetite levels or appetite-related ailments.

Because they are so sweet, bananas are a very good healthy alternative to sweets, cakes and biscuits for those with a sweet tooth, and they will make almost any dish sweeter. Dried bananas have an even sweeter taste and are particularly useful in cooking; they also have a higher concentration of potassium and fibre than the fresh fruit.

Choosing and storing

Buy firm bananas, with a strong yellow colour and few brown flecks. They are a delicious raw food, will mix with most other fruits, and are a perfect snack when you're on the go. Bananas can be cooked in a number of fruit puddings and cakes, and, for this, the riper they are the better. They are also used in some savoury dishes. Keep bananas in a cool place, out of direct sunlight. Never store them in the refrigerator.

THE BENEFITS
- Energizing
- Natural antibiotic
- Good source of fibre
- Cleansing
- Mildly sedative

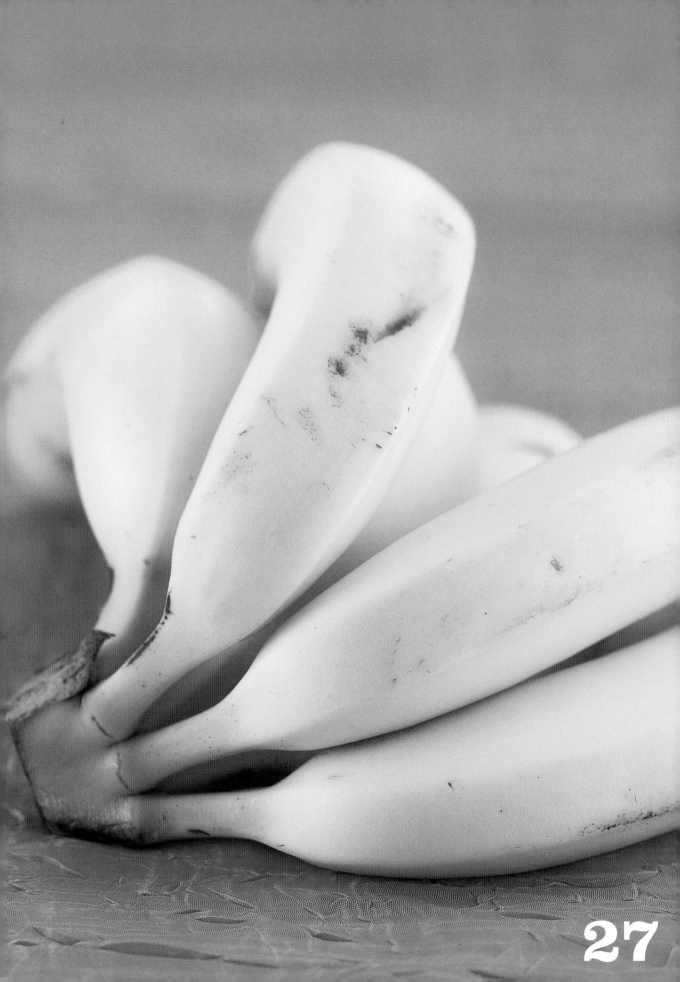

27

banana muffins with honey & yogurt

Preparation time: 10 minutes
Cooking time: 15 minutes
Makes 18

125 g (4 oz) wholemeal flour
125 g (4 oz) fine cornmeal
1 tablespoon baking powder
1 egg, beaten
2 tablespoons clear honey
150 ml (¼ pint) milk
2 bananas
150 ml (¼ pint) thick natural
   yogurt, to serve

These are ideal for breakfast or brunch on a Sunday instead of toast. Warm from the oven, they taste best spread with honey and served with thick natural yogurt. Muffins can be eaten at any time of the day; make good fillers for lunchboxes and are ideal to take on picnics.

1 Lightly grease 18 small muffin tins. If your tin is smaller, bake the muffins in batches.

2 Put the wholemeal flour, cornmeal, baking powder, beaten egg and honey into a food processor and blend together. Spoon in the milk until the mixture has a soft consistency. Peel the bananas, roughly chop the flesh and gently fold it into the muffin mixture.

3 Divide the banana mixture between the greased muffin tins and bake in the centre of a preheated oven, 180°C (350°F), Gas Mark 4, for 12-15 minutes or until risen and golden brown. Remove the muffins from the oven and allow to cool, then serve with yogurt.

jerked chicken with roasted bananas

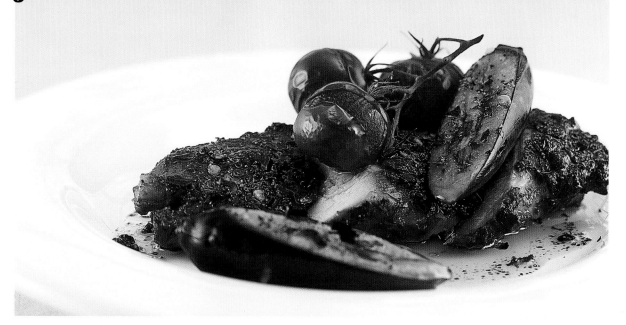

In Jamaica people roast bananas in their skins and also purée the flesh to make a highly spiced marinade for meat and fish. Both techniques are used in this detoxifying recipe.

Preparation time: 20 minutes, plus marinating
Cooking time: 30 minutes
Serves 4

5 bananas
2 tablespoons clear honey
1 tablespoon molasses
2 garlic cloves, crushed
5 tablespoons olive oil
2 teaspoons dried chilli flakes
1 teaspoon ground cumin
1 teaspoon ground coriander
4 boneless chicken breasts
1 teaspoon dried chilli flakes or
   toasted sesame seeds
sea salt and pepper
mixed salad leaves, such as
   rocket or mizuna, and roasted
   tomatoes, to serve

1 Peel one of the bananas and put it in a food processor or blender with the honey, molasses, garlic and 2 tablespoons of the olive oil and blend until smooth.

2 Heat a dry pan until hot, add the chilli flakes, cumin and coriander and toast the spices for 30-60 seconds, shaking the pan frequently. You will know they are ready when you first smell the aroma of the cumin and chilli.

3 Add the spices and salt and pepper to the banana marinade and blend until smooth. Add extra oil if the marinade seems too thick.

4 Put the chicken breasts into a shallow dish, pour the marinade over them and coat well on both sides. Cover and chill in the refrigerator for 2-6 hours.

5 Put the chicken breasts in a baking tin, skin side down, and coat well in the marinade. Roast in a preheated oven, 200°C (400°F), Gas Mark 6, for 10 minutes. Turn the chicken breasts over and brush with any remaining marinade. Cut the remaining bananas in half lengthways and put them, unpeeled, in the baking tin beside the chicken.

6 Sprinkle the bananas with the remaining oil and the chilli flakes or sesame seeds and cook for 15-20 minutes or until the chicken is cooked through and the bananas are soft. Serve the chicken thickly sliced, with the roasted bananas still in their skins, roasted tomatoes and mixed salad leaves.

beans & lentils (p

This extensive and nutritious family of foods includes red, green and brown lentils, red, white and black kidney beans, chickpeas and haricot, aduki, flageolet, black-eyed, mung and butter beans. The versatile soya bean is treated separately on page 113.

Good value foods

Pulses are widely available, easy to store and cook, and generally inexpensive. They are very useful sources of protein, making them an excellent alternative to meat for vegetarians and for those wanting to reduce animal fats in their diet. They are also a good form of carbohydrate, with slow-release sugars. These do not send a sudden rush of sugar into the blood, causing a yo-yoing of energy levels and, often, mood swings. They give a constant source of energy throughout the day, with a steadying effect on blood sugar levels.

The oestrogen connection

Pulses contain phytoestrogens, or plant oestrogens, which occur naturally in certain plants and mimic female hormones. These phytoestrogens have a stabilizing effect on the menstrual cycle and are believed to be highly beneficial in regulating erratic periods, tackling PMS and relieving menopausal symptoms, such as hot flushes and night sweats. They are used increasingly as an alternative to HRT (hormone replacement therapy). There is also increasing evidence that pulses lower breast cancer risks and protect against fibroids (benign tumours in the uterus, most common in childless, pre-menopausal women over the age of 35).

Mineral wealth

Most pulses are high in minerals, including iron, potassium, selenium, calcium, manganese, magnesium and folic acid. They are excellent intestinal cleansers and increase the friendly bacteria of the gut that aid digestion. They are a staple of detoxifying diets and also cleanse the blood and lower cholesterol. Lentils contain a number of B vitamins which help to stabilize

blood pressure. They are also anti-inflammatory, especially for rheumatoid arthritis. Chickpeas are beneficial for those with kidney stones.

Choosing and storing

It is advisable to buy pulses in a store with a quick turnover; the older they are, the longer they will take to cook. Store in airtight containers, in a cool, preferably dark cupboard, and don't expose them to direct sunlight, which leaches nutrients. Use within six months. Always pick over pulses, particularly lentils, for stones and rinse them before cooking. Different pulses have different soaking and cooking times, but you can speed up the soaking process by bringing them to the boil for a few minutes, then leaving them to stand for an hour before cooking. You can also use a pressure cooker. Cook pulses in unsalted water and reserve the liquid as a basis for soup and stocks. Kidney beans must be boiled for 15 minutes to neutralize toxins, always refer to packet instructions before cooking.

Some beans are available in canned form, but these are not so nutritious as the dried varieties and often contain sugar – notably 'baked' (haricot) beans – so always check the labels carefully. Finally, some people find that pulses bring an unwanted side-effect – flatulence. This can be alleviated by mixing them with parsley, fennel, ginger or cayenne pepper.

The Benefits
- **Improve intestinal health**
- **Reduce menopausal symptoms, PMS and risk of fibroids**
- **Lower risk of breast cancer**
- **Lower cholesterol**
- **Alleviate kidney stones**
- **Relieve rheumatoid arthritis**

ulses)

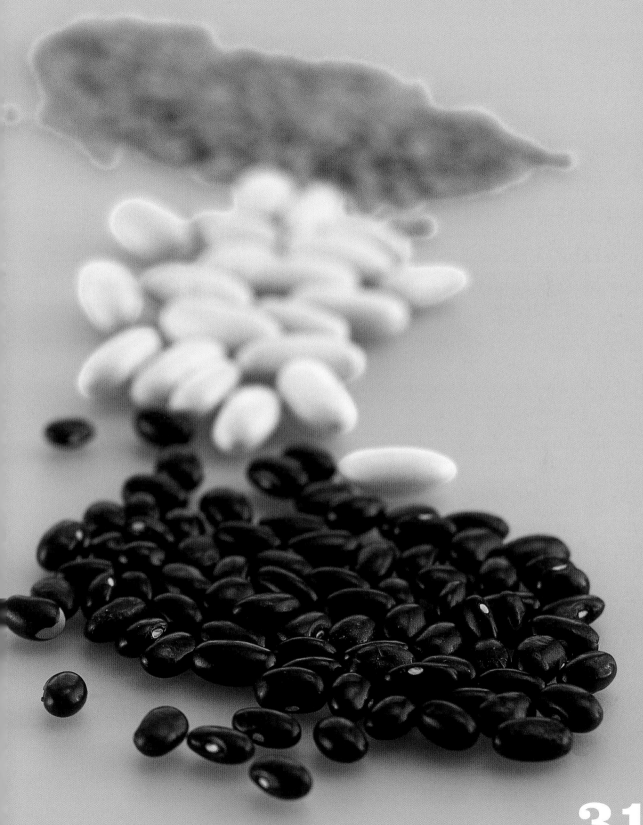

cannellini bean mash on bruschetta with rocket

Preparation time: 15 minutes
Cooking time: 6–8 minutes
Serves 4–6

2 x 400 g (13 oz) cans organic
    cannellini beans, drained
    and rinsed
2 tablespoons chopped parsley
5 tablespoons olive oil, plus
    extra for drizzling
2 garlic cloves, crushed
1 small red onion, finely chopped
2 teaspoons thyme leaves
1 teaspoon lemon juice
½ teaspoon pepper
6 maple-cured bacon rashers
    (optional)
12 slices thick ciabatta bread
12 black olives
12 cherry tomatoes
handful of rocket leaves

This delicious white kidney bean mash, which is loaded with garlic and thyme, can be piled on to ciabatta bread to make a hearty lunchtime snack, or, for a more substantial protein-rich meal, the purée can be served with roasted cod or hake or poached chicken. Dried white kidney beans can be used as an alternative; follow packet instructions for soaking and cooking times.

1 Put the beans into a bowl with the parsley and crush them to a rustic mash with the back of a spoon or a potato masher. Heat the olive oil slowly in a small pan with the crushed garlic and red onion for 1–2 minutes or until the garlic is just turning a light golden brown. Do not cook any longer or the garlic will burn and the oil will become bitter.

2 Remove the pan from the heat, add the thyme and leave to infuse for 5 minutes. Add the garlic oil, thyme and onion mixture to the bean mash, together with the lemon juice and pepper. Fork the oil through the mash.

3 Cook the bacon, if using, under a preheated grill until crisp, turning once. Add the slices of ciabatta bread and toast on both sides until golden. While the bread is still warm, spoon the bean mash on to the bruschetta and drizzle with extra olive oil if liked. Top the beans with the crisp bacon, a few black olives, cherry tomatoes and rocket leaves. Serve immediately.

oven-baked falafel & red onion salad with markouk bread

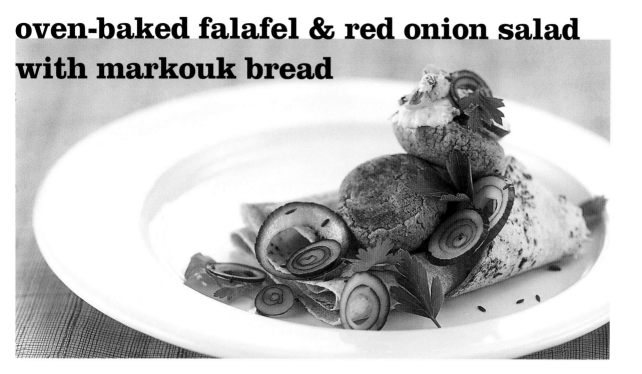

Preparation time: 25 minutes, plus chilling
Cooking time: 22 minutes
Serves 4–6

2 x 400 g (13 oz) cans organic chickpeas
3 garlic cloves, crushed
2 teaspoons ground coriander
1 small onion, finely chopped
4 tablespoons chopped coriander
1 large egg, beaten
2 tablespoons groundnut or vegetable oil
1 red onion
handful of coriander leaves
handful of flat leaf parsley
1 teaspoon cumin seeds
2 tablespoons lemon juice
150 ml (¼ pint) thick natural yogurt
½ cucumber, grated and drained
sea salt and pepper
8 sheets Middle Eastern (markouk) flat bread, to serve

Falafel are an Israeli speciality that are normally deep-fried. Here they are lightly brushed with oil and baked in the oven until crisp. The red onion salad accompanies them to add crunch and a typical Middle Eastern sweet onion flavour.

1 Put the chickpeas, crushed garlic, ground coriander, chopped onion and coriander leaves into a food processor or blender and blend until well mixed and a fairly smooth purée.

2 Beat the egg with salt and pepper, add to the chickpea mixture and blend well. Take walnut-size pieces of the mixture and press into 24 flat patties. Arrange on a lightly greased baking tray and chill for 4 hours or overnight.

3 Brush the falafel with the oil and bake in a preheated oven, 200°C (400°F), Gas Mark 6, for 20 minutes, turning once.

4 Meanwhile, thinly slice the red onion and place it in a bowl with the coriander and parsley leaves.

5 Heat a dry pan and toast the cumin seeds. Add them to the red onion salad with the lemon juice and leave to stand for 10 minutes.

6 Mix the yogurt with the grated cucumber and salt and pepper. When the falafel are cooked, wrap them in the Middle Eastern bread with some of the red onion salad and a large spoonful of cucumber and yogurt.

beetroot

This is the Cinderella of the vegetable world. Scorned by association with the bottles of pickled slices soaked in sugar and vinegar that lurk at the back of kitchen cupboards, it is finally enjoying a revival as the fresh vegetable begins to appear on the supermarket shelves.

Beet benefits

Beetroot has such powerful and wide-ranging benefits, it is difficult to know where to begin. It is one of the great cleansers and immune system strengtheners, having a beneficial effect on the entire system. It has a very high antioxidant content and helps fight off infection. It works in a profound way to stimulate the circulatory system, helping to build up red blood cells, cleansing and strengthening the blood, which enables it to carry nutrients throughout the body and overcome anaemia. In eastern Europe its blood purifying properties are so highly regarded that it is even used in leukaemia treatments. Beetroots' iron and natural sugar content strengthens and energizes the body, and it is also believed to improve memory and concentration. Whilst beetroot is naturally sweet in taste it is suprisingly low in calories.

Beneficial vitamins and minerals include beta-carotene (which metabolizes within the body to vitamin A), vitamins B6 and C, folic acid, manganese, calcium, magnesium, iron, potassium and phosphorus. It is high in carbohydrate.

Vital organs

Beetroot also protects many of the body's vital organs. It strengthens the functioning of the kidneys, gall bladder and liver, and works powerfully against kidney stones. It is a natural anti-inflammatory agent and so can help to soothe allergic reactions.

Because of its links with the blood, beetroot can be very helpful in alleviating menstrual problems, particularly anaemia caused by very heavy periods, and also as a regulator for the cycle. It also benefits menopausal problems.

Beetroot contains important antioxidants which help the body to ward off disease. The lymphatic system – the body's primary defence against infection – is strengthened by beetroot, especially when taken as a juice.

Choosing, storing and using

Choose firm, red-purple beetroot with unbroken skins, preferably organic ones with their tops still on. The leaves should be green and fresh looking. You can cook beetroot in a number of dishes; it is usually boiled, but can also be eaten raw, grated or thinly sliced, in salads. It is very common in Russian and eastern European recipes.

The juice is one of the most powerful that you can make and, if you mix it with that of other vegetables, such as carrot, spinach and cabbage, it produces one of the best all-round health cocktails you will ever find. Many people who don't like the idea of eating beetroot, enjoy the sweet, earthy taste of the juice, especially when drunk with other, more peppery or bitter vegetable juices. There are extra nutrients in the beet tops – so make sure you use the leaves, too, when you juice. The only disadvantage is that beetroot juice can stain clothes and table linen, so be careful when preparing, serving and eating.

The Benefits
- **Cleanses and detoxifies**
- **Strengthens immune and circulation systems**
- **Strengthens blood and fights anaemia**
- **Fights infection, inflammation, kidney stones**
- **Energizes and balances**

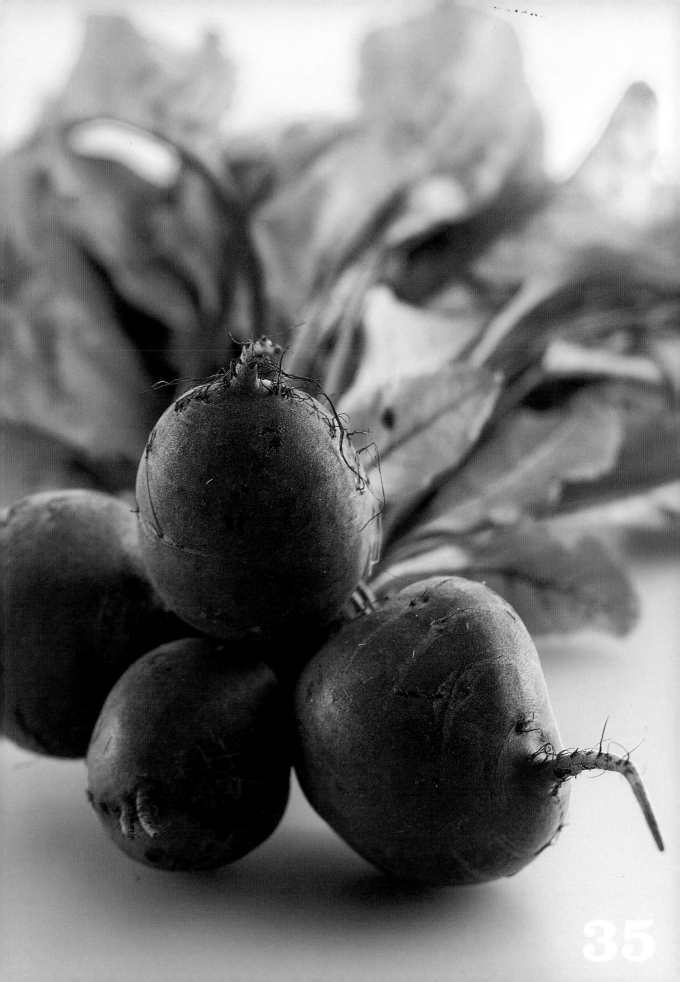

borscht with apple

Preparation time: 15 minutes
Cooking time: 40 minutes
Serves 4–6

500 g (1 lb) raw beetroot
1 small fennel bulb
600 ml (1 pint) apple juice
1 teaspoon thyme leaves
4 tablespoons lemon juice
1 tablespoon chopped chives
sea salt and pepper
soda bread, to serve

Beetroot has an amazing colour and is packed with iron, beta-carotene and folic acid. For the deepest colour and the finest flavour organic beets are best; here they team well with apple in an adaptation of the traditional Russian soup. Some like to add soured cream just before serving; if the soup is chilled, add a spoonful of thick natural yogurt.

1 Peel the beetroot and cut the flesh into thin matchstick strips. Be careful of the juice since it stains clothes and will stain your hands as you peel away the skin and cut into the flesh. If you prefer, wear gloves while preparing.

2 Trim the fennel and cut the bulb into strips. Put the beetroot and fennel into a saucepan with 600 ml (1 pint) water and bring slowly to the boil. Cover the pan and and simmer gently for 20-30 minutes or until the vegetables are tender.

3 Add the apple juice, thyme leaves and salt and pepper and simmer for a further 10 minutes. Remove from the heat and add the lemon juice and chopped chives. Season to taste with salt and pepper and serve hot, warm or cold with soda bread.

beetroot mash with butter beans & roast cod

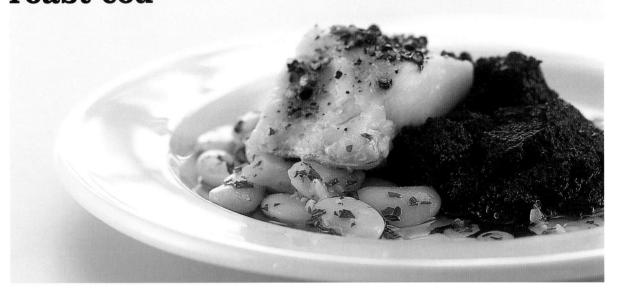

Preparation time: 25 minutes
Cooking time: 2 hours 25 minutes
Serves 4

4 x 175 g (6 oz) thick cod steaks
4 tablespoons olive oil, plus
   extra for drizzling
2 garlic cloves
400 g (13 oz) can organic
   butter beans
1 tablespoon chopped flat
   leaf parsley
sea salt and pepper
lemon wedges, to serve

Beetroot mash:
1 kg (2 lb) raw beetroot
1–2 tablespoons freshly
   grated horseradish or
   creamed horseradish

Beetroot is fabulously sweet and utterly delicious when it is just roasted simply in the oven for an hour or two, wrapped in foil. The beets can be served whole as a vegetable accompaniment to fish or meat or they can be roughly mashed to a purée.

1 Wrap each beetroot in foil and bake in a preheated oven, 200°C (400°F), Gas Mark 6, for 1–2 hours, depending on the size of the beets. They are cooked when the tip of a knife or skewer can be inserted easily into the flesh. Remove the beets from the oven, unwrap them and peel away the skins. Allow to cool.

2 Meanwhile, season the cod steaks with salt and pepper, place them in a roasting tin and drizzle with a little olive oil. Roast in the centre of the oven for 15–20 minutes or until the fish is just cooked through.

3 To make the mash, roughly chop the beetroot and place it in a food processor or blender with the horseradish, salt and pepper and blend to a coarse purée.

4 Heat the olive oil in a saucepan, add the garlic and fry gently for 30–60 seconds. Do not allow the garlic to burn. Add the butter beans and chopped parsley and toss in the hot oil for 1–2 minutes, then remove from the heat.

5 Serve the cod hot from the oven on a large spoonful or two´of beetroot mash and accompanied by the garlic butter beans and lemon wedges.

berries

Summer's cornucopia of soft fruits includes strawberries, raspberries, blackberries, blueberries, blackcurrants and redcurrants. These delicious berries are all highly protective of your immune health.

Immune protection

Some berries contain most of the essential antioxidant vitamins (A - in its beta-carotene form, C and E), while others contain them all. This makes berries particularly important for immune health, as these super-scavenger vitamins neutralize the free radicals that on a cellular level are responsible for many of the things that go wrong with our bodies. These fruits can protect not only against infections, but against more serious degenerative diseases too, as well as the problems of premature ageing.

Youth and vigour

Their high antioxidant content ensures that berries have a deep cleansing and, ultimately, anti-ageing effect. Strawberries are also thought to be beneficial for the skin - smoothing out lines and wrinkles - and for soothing arthritic inflammation.

Raspberries are a mild laxative and good, too, for indigestion. They are also beneficial for menstrual problems and, like all berries, have high levels of phytoestrogens (see page 30) and so are helpful for erratic periods, PMS and menopausal problems. Raspberry leaf tea, incidentally, is an age-old herbal remedy recommended for late pregnancy, childbirth and new mothers, as it is believed to strengthen the uterus. It is also used to treat a variety of menstrual problems, including painful cramps.

Blackcurrants, redcurrants and blueberries are excellent blood cleansers, as are blackberries, which are also extremely energizing. Blackberries and cranberries are effective at clearing congestion in the respiratory tract, as well as soothing sore throats.

Cranberries and blackcurrants are beneficial for kidney, bladder and urinary tract infections.

Many berries also contain high levels of minerals, especially calcium, magnesium and potassium. Calcium, essential for strong bones and teeth, is also necessary for the smooth functioning of the nervous system, muscles and heart. Magnesium and potassium are important, too, for a healthy heart and nervous system. These minerals, plus the traces of iron and zinc in many berries, are vital for cellular growth and health.

Choosing, storing and using

Soft fruits deteriorate rapidly so they should be eaten soon after purchase. Buy ripe fruits - organic ones if possible - checking that they are not already over-ripe. Discard any that show signs of mould. If you can buy berries freshly picked from the farm, or grow your own, these are the most nutritious and delicious tasting of all. Always remove soft fruit from plastic wrapping as soon as you get home. Wash it thoroughly and keep in the refrigerator until you are ready to eat it.

Soft fruit is best eaten raw. Ripe fruit should be sweet enough to eat unsweetened, but you can add a little honey and fruit juice. Serve with yogurt or ice cream. You can also make some sensational puddings from soft fruit, as well as jams.

The Benefits
- **Fibre enhances digestive health**
- **High antioxidant content protects against infection and disease**
- **Promote cellular health and renewal**
- **Blackcurrants, blackberries, redcurrants and blueberries all cleanse the blood and tone the circulation**
- **Cranberries are beneficial for kidney, bladder and urinary infections**
- **Blackcurrants can be beneficial for respiratory infections**

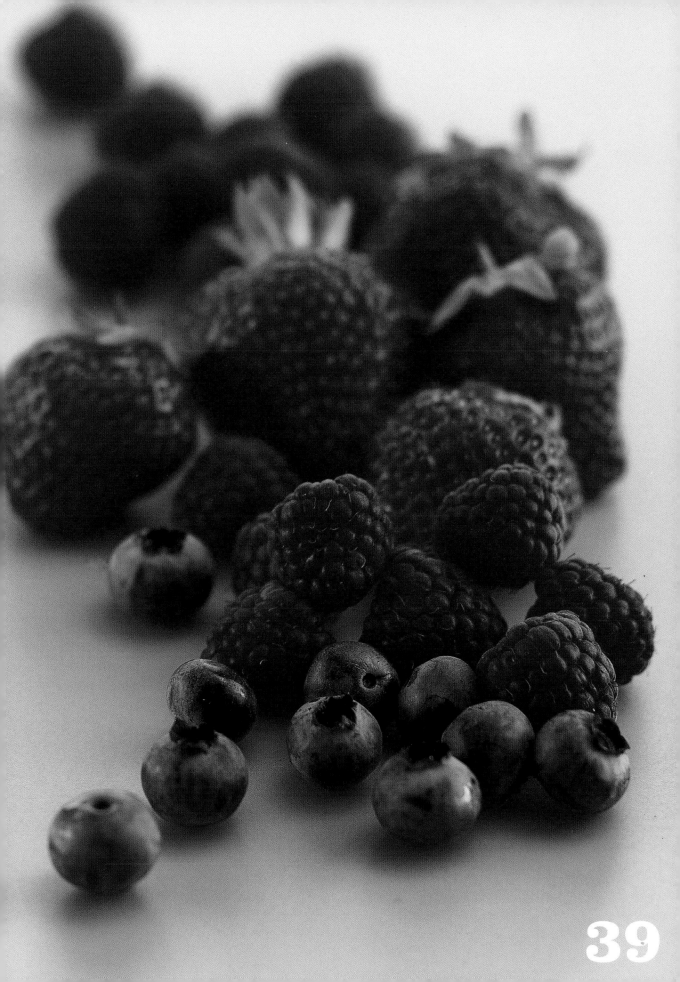

strawberry & vanilla soup

**Preparation time: 10 minutes,
    plus marinating**
Serves 4

500 g (1 lb) strawberries
1 small vanilla pod
450 ml (¾ pint) apple or
    cranberry juice
1–2 tablespoons clear honey
mint sprigs, to serve

Fresh strawberries have a wonderful aroma and nutritive content. This no-cook soup retains the heat-soluble vitamins and makes a refreshing finish to lunch or supper. It can even be eaten for breakfast with a large spoonful of yogurt and an oatcake.

1 Hull the strawberries and roughly chop the berries. Cut the vanilla pod in half lengthways and scrape out the seeds with the tip of a knife.

2 Put the strawberries into a bowl with the vanilla seeds and the empty vanilla pod, add 150 ml (¼ pint) of the apple or cranberry juice, cover and leave to stand for 1 hour for the flavours to infuse.

3 Remove and discard the vanilla pod. Put the strawberries, apple or cranberry marinade and honey into a food processor or blender and blend until smooth. Add the remaining apple or cranberry juice and blend once more. Chill until you are ready to serve

4 Serve cold in large bowls topped with mint sprigs.

lingonberry & orange fruit salad

Preparation time: 15 minutes,
   plus cooling and chilling
Cooking time: 10 minutes
Serves 4–6

125 g (4 oz) lingonberries or
   cranberries
150 ml (¼ pint) orange or apple
   juice
1–3 tablespoons clear honey
4 large oranges
1 tablespoon orange liqueur
   (optional)

To serve:
thick yogurt or fromage frais
oatmeal biscuits

Serve this tangy and refreshing fruit salad as a dessert or for breakfast. Lingonberries are a small red berry grown in Scandinavia; they are available in some large supermarkets. Alternatively, use cranberries and add extra honey to sweeten them.

1 Put the berries into a saucepan with the orange, or apple, juice and poach very gently for 10 minutes.

2 Remove from the heat and sweeten with the honey to taste. Leave to cool.

3 Peel the oranges and cut away the thick white pith. Thickly slice or segment the fruit and place in a bowl.

4 Pour the poached berries and juice over the oranges and chill in the refrigerator for 30 minutes, to allow the flavours to mingle.

5 Sprinkle the orange liqueur, if using, over the fruit and serve with thick yogurt or fromage frais and oatmeal biscuits.

A fresh berry salad can be elevated to a more elegant dessert with a spoonful of yogurt or fromage frais and a sprinkling of sugar, which is grilled until bubbling. Any fresh summer berries can be used; their vitamin content remains unaltered by the heat of the grill. The top of the yogurt or fromage frais will be warm with a touch of sweetness.

Preparation time: 10 minutes,
    plus chilling
Cooking time: 2 minutes
Serves 4

250 g (8 oz) blueberries
250 g (8 oz) raspberries
350 ml (12 fl oz) thick Greek
    yogurt or fromage frais
4–6 tablespoons soft dark brown
    muscovado or molasses sugar

1 Mix together the blueberries and raspberries and divide between 4 heatproof dishes or place in 1 large dish.

2 Spoon the yogurt or fromage frais over the berries and smooth the top. At this point the puddings can be returned to the refrigerator to chill overnight or until required.

3 Sprinkle the sugar over the yogurt or fromage frais in an even layer and place the dishes on a baking tray. Grill under a preheated grill, close to the heat, for 1-2 minutes or until the sugar has melted and is bubbling in places. Serve immediately.

blueberry & raspberry brûlée

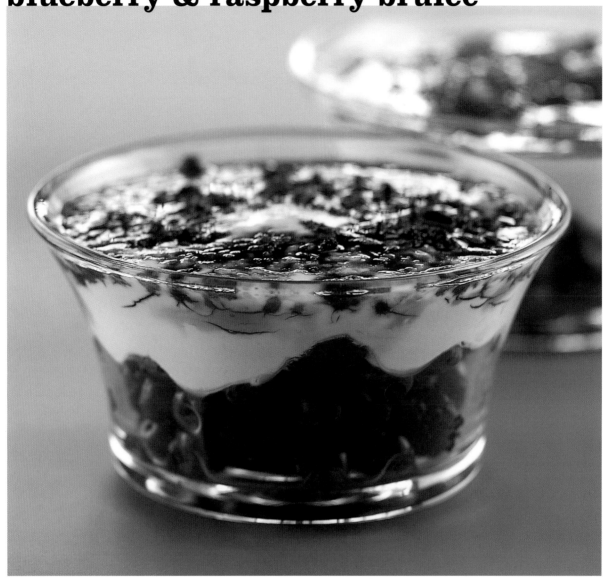

Their high antioxidant content ensures that berries have a deep cleansing and, ultimately, anti-ageing effect.

broccoli

This is a truly miraculous vegetable. Broccoli is a powerhouse of antioxidants with an unusually high protein content, while gram for gram it has half the fibre of wholemeal bread, with only a tenth of its calories.

Immune warrior

Broccoli has a high vitamin and mineral content containing beta-carotene, vitamin A, vitamin C, iron and zinc, together with a range of B vitamins and folic acid. It is profoundly strengthening for the immune system and has now been recognized by many medical authorities as a major force in combating cancer of the bowel. This is because broccoli contains sulphuraphane, a substance which detoxifies and effectively secretes the carcinogens we are breathing in and eating all the time. It is very protective of the immune system as a whole, not only against cancer, but also against heart disease and a range of infections, particularly those affecting the respiratory system.

Deep cleansing

High in both antioxidants and fibre, broccoli is a deeply cleansing vegetable. It cleanses not only the entire digestive system, it purifies and stimulates the liver too – the body's most important organ of detoxification. This has a beneficial effect on the entire system, as when the liver is working to its full potential, the whole body functions better.

Broccoli prevents a build-up of harmful toxins within the system and you can even see the difference. When the body's toxic load is reduced, the skin visibly improves – making broccoli an excellent beauty food. Its vitamin B2 content is another beauty booster, benefiting skin, hair and nails. Vitamins B2 and B5 combine powerfully in broccoli to metabolize fats into energy, so it gives you a boost in more ways than one. Proper cooking is essential to ensure broccoli retains its beneficial nutrients.

Folic acid

As a good source of folic acid (another B vitamin), broccoli is also particularly valuable for pregnant women. Folic acid protects against spina bifida in unborn babies and strengthens the nervous systems and blood cells of mothers and babies alike. The oral contraceptive pill may also reduce folic acid levels, which can result in anaemia. Folic acid also promotes the production of serotonin, a mood-lifting chemical that is produced naturally within the body, so broccoli may also be beneficial for people suffering from depression. It is recommended that 1–3 portions of broccoli should be eaten a week.

Choosing, storing and using

Look for broccoli with a good, strong green colour. Avoid any that is starting to turn yellow or wilt. You can also, of course, buy purple sprouting broccoli, which has a loose head of florets. The stems of both types should be very firm to the touch. Eat broccoli within a day or two of purchase and until then, store in the refrigerator.

The best way to cook broccoli is to steam it. Never overcook it – it needs only a few minutes. To boil it use a small amount of water, cover the saucepan with a lid and boil for just a few minutes.

The Benefits
- **Fights bowel cancer**
- **Protects the immune system**
- **Detoxifies the digestive system and liver**
- **Protects unborn babies against risk of spina bifida**
- **Enhances mood**
- **Improves skin**

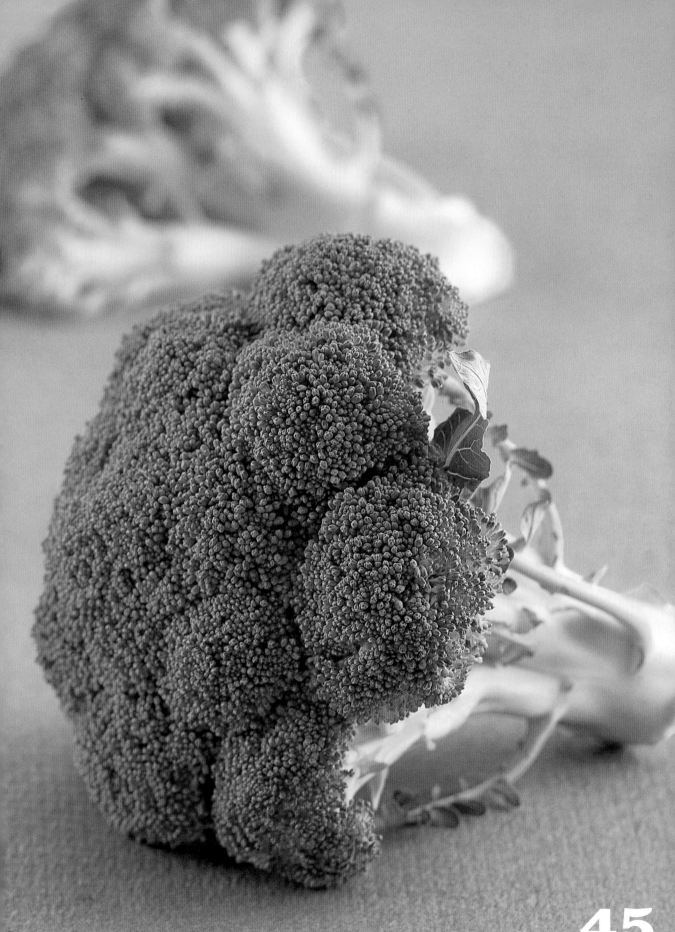

stir-fried broccoli with sesame seeds & red rice

To help retain the broccoli's nutritional content it is not cooked for long and certainly not boiled. Briefly blanched, it is then quickly stir-fried with a mix of other crunchy green vegetables. For a bonus, kombu may be added to the rice cooking water to allow the iron in the seaweed to be absorbed by the grains. This makes a good lunch or supper dish and also can be taken as a packed lunch.

Preparation time: 15 minutes
Cooking time: 35 minutes
Serves 4

500 g (1 lb) broccoli florets
125 g (4 oz) sugar snap peas
125 g (4 oz) mangetouts
250 g (8 oz) red or brown rice
10 cm (4 inch) piece of dried
   kombu seaweed (optional)
3 tablespoons groundnut oil
2–3 garlic cloves, crushed
3 tablespoons soy sauce
1 tablespoon tahini paste
1 tablespoon sesame oil
2 tablespoons sesame
   seeds, toasted
pepper

1 Bring a pan of water to the boil. Plunge the broccoli into the water for 1 minute, then remove with a slotted spoon and immediately add to a bowl of cold water to refresh and prevent any further cooking.

2 Trim the sugar snaps and mangetouts and blanch them in the boiling water for 30 seconds. Remove them from the boiling water with a slotted spoon and refresh in the bowl of cold water for 5 minutes, then drain well. Reserve the pan of vegetable water.

3 Add the red or brown rice to the pan of vegetable water with the kombu, if using, and return to the boil. Reduce the heat a little and cook at a fast simmer for 30 minutes. When the rice is just cooked and still retains a bite, drain well, reserving a little of the water, and discard the seaweed.

4 Heat the groundnut oil in a wok or large frying pan, add the garlic and cook gently, stirring constantly, for 1 minute to flavour the oil. Do not allow the garlic to burn.

5 Add the drained vegetables to the oil and stir-fry for 1-2 minutes. Mix together the soy sauce, tahini, sesame oil and 8 tablespoons of reserved vegetable water, add to the vegetables and stir-fry for a further 1 minute.

6 Remove the wok from the heat and toss the cooked red or brown rice through the vegetables. Spoon into serving bowls and top with toasted sesame seeds and black pepper. Serve immediately or chill and serve cold.

broccoli with anchovies & trottole

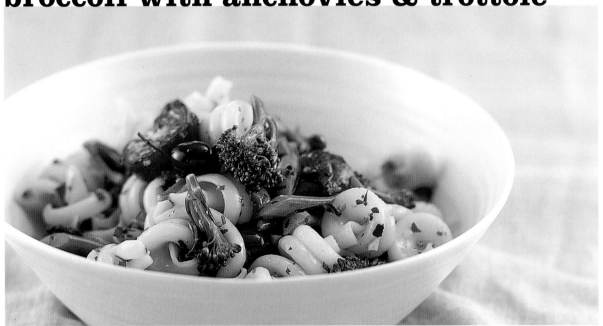

Broccoli, also known as poor man's asparagus, is packed with a cocktail of vitamins and minerals. Asparagus, kale or any green vegetable can also be used in this recipe: prepare them in exactly the same way, briefly blanching the vegetables to retain as many minerals and vitamins as possible.

Preparation time: 15 minutes
Cooking time: 20 minutes
Serves 4

350 g (12 oz) trottole, orecchetti or penne pasta
8 tablespoons olive oil
4 garlic cloves, crushed
6 anchovy fillets
10 cherry tomatoes, halved and roasted
250 g (8 oz) broccoli, stalk and florets, roughly chopped
3 tablespoons capers
3 tablespoons chopped parsley
½ teaspoon pepper
3 tablespoons basil leaves
8–10 black olives, pitted

1 Bring a large saucepan of water to the boil, add the pasta and boil for 8–12 minutes or until the pasta is al dente and still has a bite.

2 Heat 2 tablespoons of the oil in a large saucepan, add the garlic and heat gently for 1–2 minutes to release the flavour. Do not allow the garlic to burn or over-brown. Add the anchovy fillets and roasted tomatoes to the oil and cook gently for 2–3 minutes, stirring occasionally. The juice from the tomato will ooze out and the anchovy fillets will disintegrate into the oil.

3 Put the broccoli into a bowl, cover with boiling water and leave to stand for 2 minutes. Drain well and transfer to a bowl of cold water to refresh and stop any further cooking.

4 Add the broccoli to the pan of flavoured oil with the capers and coat in the oil. Drain the pasta and add to the pan with the chopped parsley and toss together.

5 Add the remaining olive oil, the pepper, basil leaves and olives and mix lightly. Serve while piping hot.

cabbage

There are three main types of cabbage – green, red and white. They are all powerful antioxidant vegetables and believed, like broccoli, to have cancer-fighting properties. Green cabbage has the highest concentration of nutrients.

Colon cleanser

When eaten raw or used as part of a fresh vegetable juice cocktail, cabbage is of particular benefit to the digestion. It detoxifies the whole digestive system, in particular the stomach and the upper colon. It soothes stomach upsets and indigestion and, taken long term as a daily juice, it helps heal stomach ulcers. It is also very helpful for anyone who suffers from constipation, as not only does it help eradicate the ailment itself by encouraging peristalsis, but it is also deeply cleansing for the colon, which can suffer from a build-up of toxins in cases of long-term constipation.

Mineral rich

Cabbage contains a number of valuable minerals. Calcium is essential for strong bones and teeth, as well as the proper functioning of the nervous system, muscles, the heart and blood clotting. Magnesium also promotes healthy muscles and nerve functioning, repairing the body on a cellular level. Potassium and phosphorus are both needed for a healthy heart and kidneys, while iodine – rarely found in land vegetables – is important for thyroid function, energy and growth.

Skin health

A powerful antioxidant (containing high levels of vitamins A, C and E) and a deep cleanser, cabbage also purifies the blood and can improve cases of oily skin prone to acne, particularly if taken as a juice. It benefits all skin types and cabbage water (the water in which cabbage has been boiled) is an age-old pick-me-up for a tired complexion. It is also traditionally believed to be a hangover cure, probably because it is such an effective cleanser of the liver, where the metabolism of alcohol begins.

Coughs and colds

Cabbage is antibacterial and boosts the immune system. Its high vitamin C content helps to build up resistance to coughs, colds and other infections, and cabbage water is also helpful in soothing coughs and clearing the head and bronchial passages. Cabbage water works particularly well if you add a pinch of ginger or cayenne pepper to it.

Choosing, storing and using

Green cabbages should have a firm heart and a good strong colour. As the outer leaves often have the most nutrients, choose ones with undamaged outer leaves if possible. Even if they are damaged, they can still be used for cooking or juicing. Steam cabbage for 4–6 minutes rather than boiling it.

Red and white cabbages are harder and more tightly furled than green ones. Look for a strong colour with the outer leaves intact. Red and white cabbages can both be eaten raw in salads or cooked, red cabbage being particularly popular in eastern European dishes. Like green cabbages, they make very effective juices, but should always be mixed with something sweeter (such as carrot or beetroot), as cabbage juice has a strong, bitter taste.

Use all cabbages as soon as possible after purchase, store in the refrigerator and wash thoroughly before eating or cooking.

The Benefits
- Has anti-cancer properties
- Boosts the immune system
- Fights bacteria
- Improves skin
- Tones liver and digestive system
- Improves digestive function
- Heals stomach ulcers

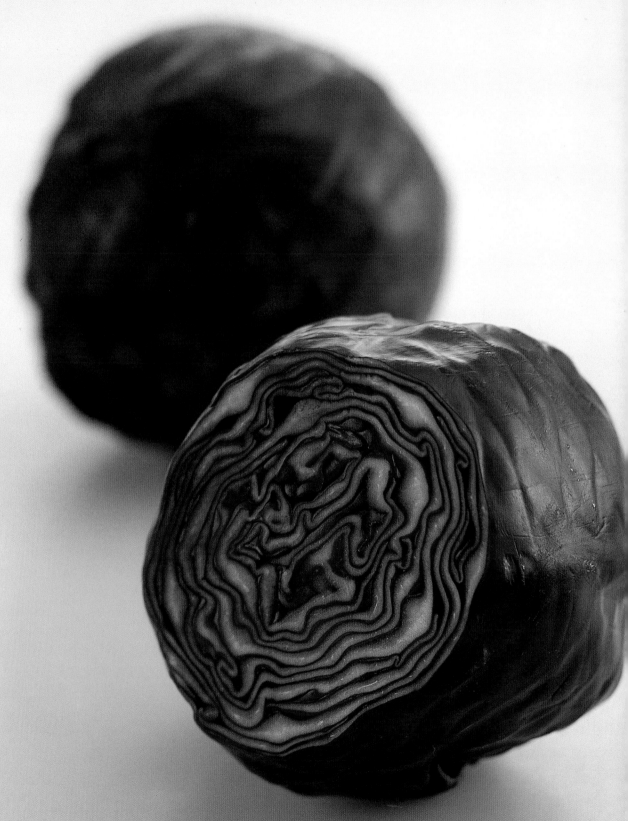

oriental cabbage rolls
with wakame broth

A main meal in one large bowl. These cabbage leaves filled with brown rice are simmered gently in a flavoured seaweed stock, retaining all the goodness in the broth. The addition of the kombu and arame seaweeds boosts the iron, calcium and potassium levels.

Preparation time: 25 minutes, plus soaking
Cooking time: 1 hour
Serves 4

15 g (½ oz) dried black ear fungus or shiitake mushrooms
8 large Savoy cabbage leaves, washed well
75 g (3 oz) brown rice
10 cm (4 inch) piece of dried kombu seaweed
3 tablespoons groundnut or vegetable oil
3 garlic cloves, crushed
5 cm (2 inch) piece of fresh root ginger, peeled and grated
1 tablespoon chopped coriander
1.2 litres (2 pints) vegetable stock
8 pearl onions or tiny shallots
2 tablespoons dried wakame seaweed
2 tablespoons mirin
large handful of coriander leaves
2 teaspoons sesame oil
10 cm (4 inch) piece of daikon or white radish (optional)
1 small fresh red chilli (optional)
pepper

1 Put the black ear fungus or dried shiitake mushrooms into a bowl, cover with 300 ml (½ pint) boiling water and leave to stand for 20 minutes to swell. Remove the mushrooms from the water and chop finely. Strain the mushroom water and reserve.

2 Meanwhile, cut the central stem out of the cabbage leaves and place the leaves in a large bowl. Pour 300 ml (½ pint) boiling water over them and blanch for 1 minute or until they are soft and pliable.

3 Remove the cabbage leaves from the boiling water, reserving the now green water, and refresh the leaves under running cold water, then drain. Add the cabbage water to the mushroom water.

4 Put the rice into a pan of cold water with the kombu seaweed and bring to the boil. Reduce the heat and simmer for 35 minutes. When the rice is cooked but still retains some bite, drain it well and discard the kombu.

5 Heat the oil in a small pan, add the garlic and heat gently, to cook the garlic and release its flavour into the oil.

6 Add the hot oil to the cooked rice with the chopped fungus or shiitake mushrooms, grated ginger and chopped coriander. Season with pepper.

7 Spread one of the cabbage leaves out flat and place a large spoonful of the rice at the stalk end. Fold over the sides and roll up the leaf into a fat cigar shape. Secure with string or a cocktail stick. Repeat with the remaining cabbage leaves and rice.

8 Put the vegetable stock in a saucepan with the reserved vegetable water, pearl onions or tiny shallots and wakame seaweed and simmer gently for 10 minutes. Add the mirin, pepper to taste and the cabbage rolls and continue to simmer gently for a further 10 minutes.

9 Remove the string or cocktail sticks from the cabbage rolls and serve in large bowls with the broth spooned over them. Add a handful of coriander leaves and a sprinkling of sesame oil.

10 Finely grate the daikon or radish and finely chop the red chilli and offer both with the soup. Eat the broth while hot, sprinkling it with daikon and chilli if liked.

red cabbage slaw

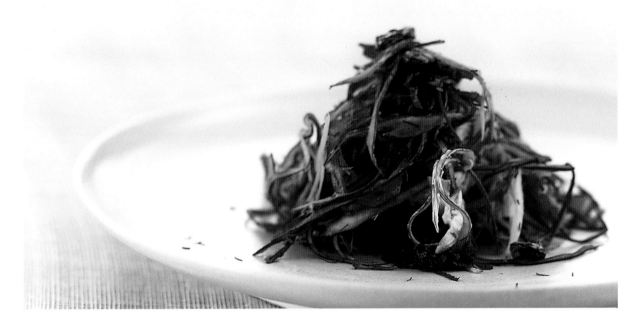

**Preparation time: 20 minutes,
plus marinating**

Serves 4–6

500 g (1 lb) red cabbage
1 red onion
1 raw beetroot
2 carrots
1 fennel bulb
2 tablespoons chopped parsley
   or dill
75 g (3 oz) raisins or sultanas
6 tablespoons thick
   natural yogurt
1 tablespoon cider or white
   wine vinegar
2 teaspoons sweet German
   mustard or Dijon mustard
1 teaspoon clear honey
1 garlic clove, crushed
sea salt and pepper
rye or sourdough bread, to serve

This is a very vivid version of a white cabbage coleslaw. The red cabbage, red onion and beetroot will colour the yogurt dressing a bright pink, while the mustard and vinegar will give the dressing a kick. Add honey and mustard according to your taste, and feel free to remove and substitute any of the vegetables. Serve as a side salad with cold meats or with roasted or sautéed fish, chicken, beef or lamb.

1 Trim the stalk end of the red cabbage and very finely shred the cabbage. Cut the red onion in half and slice it thinly. Peel the beetroot and carrots and cut them both into very thin matchsticks or grate coarsely. Halve the fennel bulb and shred it finely.

2 Put all the prepared vegetables, chopped parsley or dill and raisins or sultanas into a large bowl and toss them with your hands to combine the different vegetables.

3 Mix the yogurt with the vinegar, mustard, honey, garlic, a pinch of salt and plenty of pepper. Pour this dressing over the slaw and mix well. Leave to marinate for at least 1 hour and serve with rye or sourdough bread.

carrots

The humble carrot is one of the great detoxifying foods. It not only cleanses but it also regulates imbalances in the body. Even the story about carrots helping you see in the dark turns out to possibly be true.

Liver liberator

Carrots have a powerfully cleansing effect on the liver, the body's most important organ of detoxification, which, in turn, improves the functioning of all the related systems. They also strengthen and tone the liver function, especially in juice form. However, don't drink more than three glasses a day of carrot cocktails, using no more than two carrots each time, and mixing them with other vegetables or apple. Too much carrot juice and your skin starts to turn orange.

Beta-carotene

Carrots are a storehouse of beta-carotene, which the body converts into vitamin A, boosting the immune system, protecting and strengthening the respiratory and digestive systems, and building strong teeth, hair and bones. Beta-carotene has a healing effect on the skin, especially in cases of eczema, dermatitis and acne, and improves the complexion if taken as a juice with apple. Beta-carotene is believed to lead to improved night vision and healthy eyes.

Energy release

Carrots contain natural sugars, which they release slowly into the body to give sustained energy, rather than the sudden burst that you get from refined sugars. They work best when eaten raw. They are an excellent restorative food, especially as a soup, for anyone who is convalescing or generally run down.

A fortifying vegetable

Because carrots contain both vitamin C and beta-carotene in large quantities, they are at the forefront of resisting disease and strengthening immunity. They are believed to benefit a wide range of ailments, including respiratory infections, digestive problems and ulcers.

They also offer protection against the risk of various forms of cancer. They have a long folk remedy tradition of helping with conditions specific to women, including regulating menstruation and improving the flow of breast milk in nursing mothers, which may be linked to their high calcium content.

Carrots have an excellent effect on the blood, building up the red corpuscles, improving circulation and increasing haemoglobin. They are also believed to give protection against diseases of the heart and arteries. If you eat carrots daily, they will, over time, reduce your cholesterol levels too.

Choosing, storing and using

Buy organic carrots with a strong colour and their tops and tails still on, especially for juicing, as you can include the leaves. The leaves are often a good indicator of freshness, so look for green leaves that are not wilting or yellowed. Store in the refrigerator and eat as soon as possible after purchase.

Scrub carrots well before you use them, but if possible try not to peel them. Carrots are best eaten raw by themselves or in salads, but they are also a versatile cooked vegetable.

The Benefits
- May lower risk of cancer
- Boost the immune system
- Soothe respiratory and digestive problems
- Help to heal ulcers
- Strengthen teeth, hair, bones
- Benefit lactating women
- Improves skin
- Detoxify the liver
- Promote healthy blood cells, heart and circulation

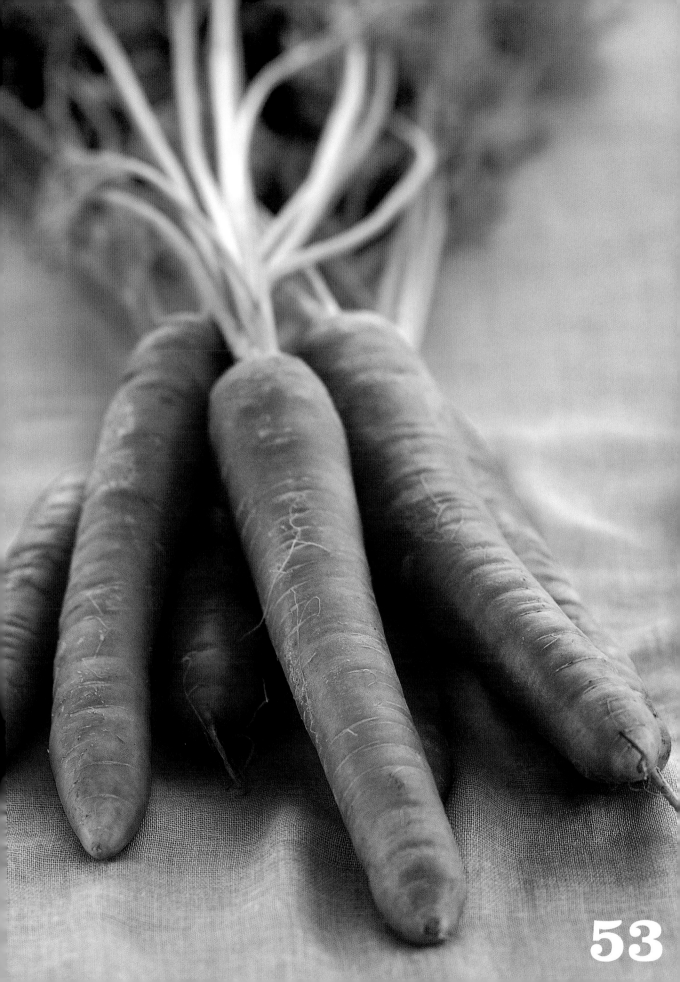

carrot, daikon & orange salad

Preparation time: 20 minutes
Serves 4–6

500 g (1 lb) carrots
250 g (8 oz) daikon or white
    radish
1 large orange
1 lemon or lime
3 tablespoons groundnut oil or
    olive oil
2 tablespoons sunflower seeds
handful of roughly
    torn watercress
sea salt and pepper

This basic salad can be made, dressed and left to chill in the refrigerator for an hour or two, but add the watercress only just before serving. For the optimum nutritive value, it would be best to prepare and eat the salad straightaway.

1 Scrub the carrots, trim the stalk end and, if they are old carrots, peel them thinly. Thinly peel the daikon radish.

2 Holding each carrot or daikon lengthways in your hand grate it on the largest holes of a grater, running the vegetables along their length against the grater. This will give you long strands. Put the grated vegetables into a bowl and toss together.

3 Scrub the orange and lemon or lime well, then finely grate the rind and add it to the salad. Toss through the vegetable strands.

4 Squeeze the orange and lemon or lime and mix the juice with the oil, salt and pepper; pour the dressing over the salad and toss together. Add the sunflower seeds and torn watercress, toss once more and serve immediately.

carrot tagine with dates & apricots

Preparation time: 20 minutes
Cooking time: 30 minutes
Serves 4–6

3 sweet white onions, sliced
2 tablespoons groundnut oil
5 cm (2 inch) piece of fresh root
   ginger, peeled and chopped
1 cinnamon stick
1 teaspoon ground cumin
1 teaspoon ground coriander
pinch of cayenne pepper
750 g (1½ lb) carrots
300 ml (½ pint) vegetable stock
1 tablespoon chilli paste (harissa)
2 tablespoons clear honey
125 g (4 oz) dates
125 g (4 oz) dried apricots
4 tablespoons lemon juice
sea salt and pepper
250 g (8 oz) couscous
2 tablespoons chopped mint
2 lemons, quartered, to serve
coriander leaves, to garnish

Cooking together carrots, dried apricots and fresh dates in a mildly spiced broth gives them a delicious aromatic flavour and means much of their nutritive value is retained in the broth. Serve with couscous, bulgar wheat or millet.

1 Briefly fry the onions in the oil until transparent. Add the fresh ginger, cinnamon stick, cumin, coriander and cayenne pepper and fry for 1 further minute.

2 Cut the carrots into 5 cm (2 inch) pieces or batons. Put them in a steamer over the stock and steam for 8-10 minutes or until tender. Remove the carrots, set aside and keep warm.

3 Add the chilli paste, honey, dates, apricots and lemon juice to the stock and simmer for 10 minutes or until the dates are tender and the sauce reduced and thick. Add the steamed carrots to the stock, season with salt and pepper and cover with a lid. Remove from the heat and leave to stand for 5 minutes.

4 Put the couscous into a large bowl and pour enough boiling water over the grains to cover them, plus 1.5 cm (¾ inch). Leave to stand for 10 minutes, then fluff the grains with a fork. Mix the chopped mint into the couscous. Serve the carrot tagine on a bed of couscous with the quartered lemons and coriander leaves.

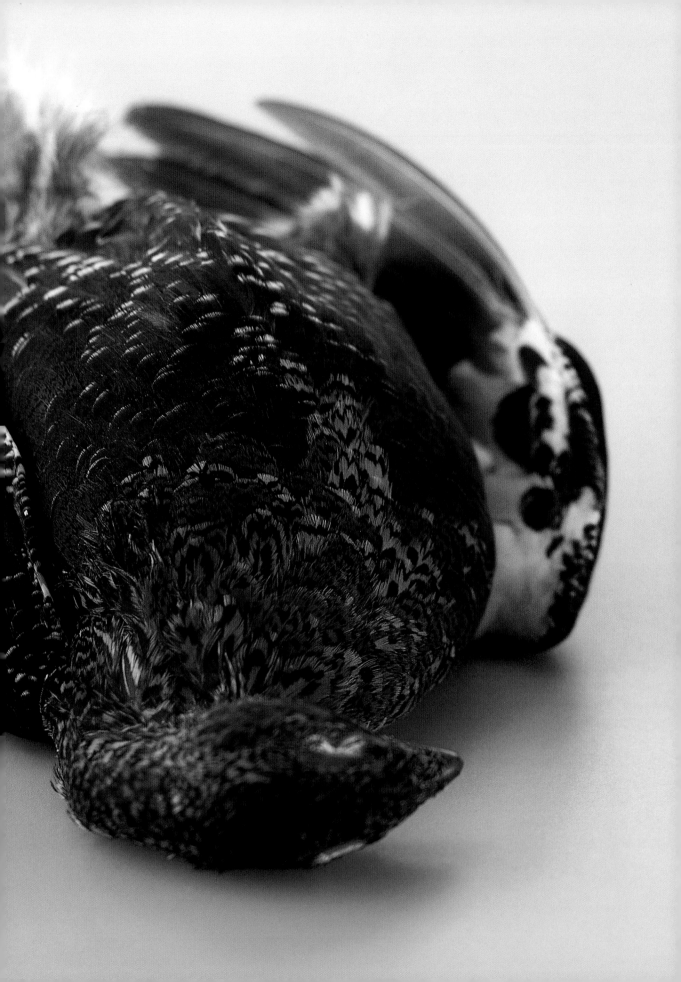

game

The term game covers various animals and birds that live in the wild and so are not subjected to the barrage of antibiotics, growth supplements and dubious farming practices suffered by most farm animals.

Lean and mean

Game includes venison, pheasant, duck, partridge and quail. These creatures are free to move around and so they acquire less fat than their farmed equivalents. This is even true of duck; though naturally inclined to be fatty, wild duck is a lot less so than the farmed variety. This means that the high fat content of farmed meat, with all its associated health problems, and the risks of passing on chemicals used in modern farming are immediately reduced.

Building blocks

Game provides a lean and nutritious form of animal protein that contains all the essential amino acids needed to build new tissues, blood, hormones and enzymes. The body uses them to repair and rebuild cells and strengthen the immune system. While an excessive intake of animal protein is associated with numerous degenerative diseases, eating game once or twice a week can be very beneficial.

Vital minerals

Selenium, zinc and iron are essential for many body processes and high levels of all these minerals are found in game. Selenium is an important antioxidant and is believed to play a vital role in protecting against heart disease and cancer. It detoxifies the liver and improves its function, which strengthens the immune system. It improves tissue strength and elasticity and plays a pivotal role in sex hormones.

Zinc is another powerful antioxidant that is vital for cellular growth and renewal. It, too, improves both liver and hormone function. It is necessary for growth, healing wounds and building resistance to infection. A high zinc intake is important for women taking oral contraceptives and for those who take diuretics.

Iron is an important mineral. It is needed for healthy blood and a lack of it can cause anaemia, particularly if you are pregnant or have heavy periods. It promotes growth and normal muscle and brain function and helps metabolize protein. Iron from animal sources is easiest to absorb.

B vitamins

Game provides all the important B vitamins, vital for the processing of food into energy. Deficiency in this group of vitamins is increasingly regarded as a cause of PMS by nutritional therapists. B1 is essential for metabolizing sugar within the body and strengthens the muscles and nervous system. B2 is needed for the metabolism of proteins and benefits the skin, hair and nails. B3 helps metabolize carbohydrates and strengthens the nervous and digestive systems. B5 is also used in metabolizing energy as well as improving adrenal gland function, helping the body cope with stress. B6 metabolizes protein and promotes production of red blood cells and antibodies, and improves the nervous and immune systems. B12 is important for iron metabolism and a healthy nervous system.

THE BENEFITS
- Repairs and regenerates cells
- Improves immune function
- Prevents anaemia
- Improves tissue strength

Choosing, storing and using

Always buy game from a reputable butcher. Young birds should be roasted slowly, while older ones are better braised or casseroled.

57

braised guinea fowl with baby carrots & celeriac mash

Guinea fowl is a very lean meat and contains plenty of iron. Because it is so lean, it dries out easily, so one of the best ways of cooking it is to braise it slowly as a pot roast with a few root vegetables. Serve with a celeriac mash, which is rich in calcium, magnesium, potassium and vitamin C.

Preparation time: 25 minutes, plus marinating
Cooking time: 1 hour
Serves 4

1 large oven-ready guinea fowl, cut into portions
7 tablespoons olive oil
2 garlic cloves, crushed
3 large thyme sprigs
2 bay leaves
6 juniper berries, roughly crushed
2 onions, finely chopped
300 ml (½ pint) vegetable stock
2 celery sticks, roughly chopped
300 g (10 oz) baby carrots, trimmed
sea salt and pepper

Celeriac mash:
1 tablespoon lemon juice
300 g (10 oz) celeriac
300 g (10 oz) potatoes
4 tablespoons crème fraîche or buttermilk
1 tablespoon chopped parsley

1 Put the guinea fowl portions into a shallow bowl. Mix together 4 tablespoons of the olive oil, the crushed garlic, thyme sprigs, bay leaves, juniper berries, salt and pepper and pour over the guinea fowl. Cover and leave to marinate for 4 hours or overnight, turning the guinea fowl once in a while.

2 Heat the remaining oil in a pan. Lift the guinea fowl portions out of the marinade, reserving the marinade. Shake off as much of the marinade as possible and brown the guinea fowl on all sides. Remove the guinea fowl from the pan, add the chopped onions and fry gently for 10–15 minutes or until golden brown.

3 Pour any remaining marinade into the pan, add the vegetable stock and chopped celery and bring to the boil. Season well with pepper, then reduce the heat and return the guinea fowl portions to the pan.

4 Cover the pan and simmer gently for 20 minutes. Remove the lid, stir carefully and add the baby carrots. Replace the lid and cook gently for a further 20 minutes.

5 Meanwhile, bring a pan of water to the boil and add the lemon juice. Peel the celeriac, quickly slice it into chunks and immediately add it to the water to prevent it from browning. Bring back to the boil and boil for 20 minutes.

6 Peel the potatoes and cut them into chunks, then add them to the celeriac and cook for a further 15-20 minutes or until both the vegetables are cooked. Drain well, then return both vegetables to the pan and mash them to a coarse purée.

7 Add the crème fraîche or buttermilk, chopped parsley, salt and pepper and mash once again. Test the pieces of guinea fowl to make sure they are cooked through. Season the sauce to taste with salt and pepper and discard the bay leaves and thyme sprigs. Serve the portions of guinea fowl on a pile of celeriac mash with the juices from the pan spooned over and around them.

spatchcocked quail with mushroom couscous

Preparation time: 20 minutes,
    plus marinating
Cooking time: 30 minutes
Serves 4

8 oven-ready quail
1 tablespoon ground cumin
2 teaspoons ground coriander
½ teaspoon chilli powder
1 teaspoon garam masala
1 garlic clove, crushed
300 ml (½ pint) thick set yogurt
4 tablespoons lemon juice
salt and pepper

Mushroom couscous:
175 g (6 oz) couscous
4–6 tablespoons olive oil
1 red onion, finely chopped
1 garlic clove, crushed
175 g (6 oz) assorted mushrooms,
    sliced
1 tablespoon chopped flat leaf
    parsley or coriander

To serve:
lemon wedges
mango chutney

Quail is one of the most delicately flavoured game birds. Roast lightly stuffed with ginger and onion, or spatchcock and grill, taking care not to overcook the delicate flesh.

1 Using a pair of sharp scissors, cut down the back of each quail to open it out, then press gently along the breastbone to flatten it.

2 Heat a dry frying pan until hot and add the ground cumin and coriander, chilli powder and garam masala. Toast the spices for 2-3 minutes, shaking the pan frequently and taking care not to burn them. If you do, start again.

3 Mix the toasted spices and the garlic into the yogurt with the lemon juice and salt and pepper to taste. Add the prepared quail to the yogurt mixture and mix well to coat. Cover the bowl and chill for 1 hour or overnight.

4 Remove the quail from the marinade and thread each one on to two pre-soaked wooden skewers, from each wing to thigh in a cross formation, to keep the birds flat as they cook.

5 Place the quail under a preheated hot grill, skin side up, and cook for 8-10 minutes on the first side and then for about 5 minutes on the second side, or until the birds are cooked through and the juices run clear. Baste the quail with any remaining marinade halfway through cooking.

6 Meanwhile, pour enough boiling water over the couscous to just cover it and set aside for 5 minutes to soak. Lightly mix the couscous with a fork to fluff up the grains and break up any lumps.

7 Heat the oil in a pan, add the chopped onion and garlic and fry for 2-3 minutes. Add the sliced mushrooms and fry quickly on all sides, shaking the pan frequently.

8 When the mushrooms are golden brown, add them to the couscous with the oil. Add the chopped parsley or coriander, season well with salt and pepper to taste and toss together with a fork.

9 Remove the wooden skewers from the quail and serve the birds on the mushroom couscous with thick lemon wedges and some mango chutney.

venison steaks
with sesame & noodles

Venison steaks are extremely lean and require very little cooking. Always undercook them, since they can be put back to cook a little longer if required, but once overcooked and dry there is no remedy. The same applies to the noodles.

Preparation time: 10 minutes, plus marinating
Cooking time: 5 minutes
Serves 4

4 x 150 g (5 oz) lean
venison steaks
3 tablespoons soy sauce
1 tablespoon oyster sauce
1 tablespoon mirin
2 garlic cloves, crushed
1 tablespoon finely grated fresh
root ginger
2 tablespoons groundnut oil
250 g (8 oz) spring greens or
choi sum
200 g (7 oz) mung bean or
buckwheat noodles
1 tablespoon sesame oil

1 Place the venison steaks in a shallow bowl. Mix 2 tablespoons of the soy sauce with the oyster sauce, mirin, garlic, ginger and groundnut oil, pour the marinade over the venison and coat thoroughly. Cover, chill and leave to marinate for 1-2 hours.

2 Place the spring greens or choi sum in a bowl and cover with boiling water. Leave for 1 minute, then drain well, reserving the vegetable water. Roughly chop the greens, set aside and keep warm.

3 Put the vegetable water into a large saucepan, add more water so the pan is half full and bring to the boil. Add the mung bean or buckwheat noodles and return the water to the boil; reduce the heat and simmer for 4-5 minutes or until the noodles are just cooked, but still firm.

4 Meanwhile, cook the venison steaks for 2 minutes on each side under a preheated grill or on a griddle, brushing them with any remaining marinade.

5 Drain the noodles the minute they are cooked. Mix together the remaining soy sauce and the sesame oil and toss through the noodles.

6 Cut the venison steaks into thick slices and serve immediately on a bed of mung bean or buckwheat noodles, topped with the wilted greens.

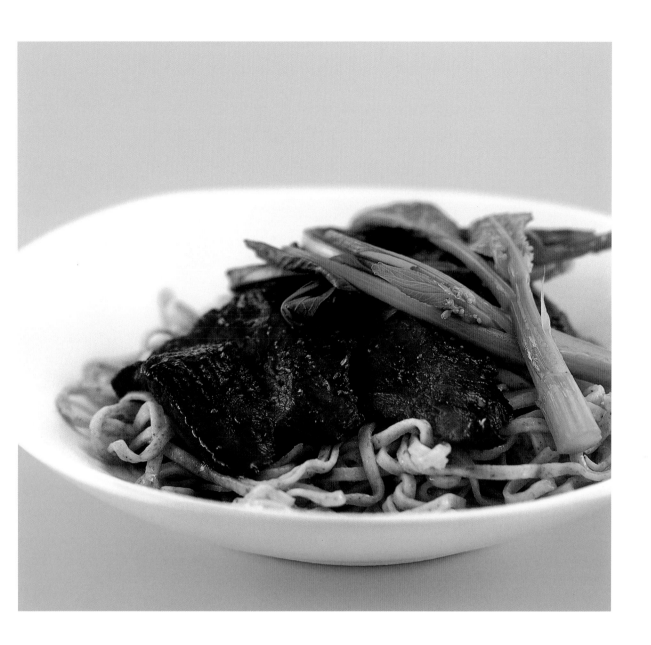

Game provides all the important B vitamins,
vital for the processing of food into energy.

garlic

Garlic is certainly miraculous in many of its properties. It is, for instance, a natural antibiotic and can stop many kinds of infections in their tracks. It also lowers cholesterol, protects the heart and promotes good circulation. Onions have many of the same health-giving qualities as garlic, though they have less potency.

A force to be reckoned with

According to the seventeenth-century herbalist Nicholas Culpeper, garlic is 'a remedy for all diseases and hurts ... It is a good preservative against and a remedy for any plague, sore or foul ulcer, takes away spots and blemishes in the skin, eases pains in the ears ... It is also held good in the jaundice, cramps, convulsions, the piles or haemorrhoids.'

Garlic is no less highly regarded today. Taken on a regular basis, it builds up high levels of resistance to infection within the immune system. It is antiviral, antibacterial and antiseptic, as well as antibiotic. This should make it a vital part of your diet at all times, but especially when you are feeling under the weather. If you take garlic in large quantities, for example, when you feel the onset of a cold, you can often fight it off before it takes a real hold. Garlic is a great detoxifier and contains a strong dose of vitamin C, as well as the antioxidant mineral selenium. Besides having these powerful antioxidants to fight free radicals, it actually leaches some of the worst toxins from the system and helps excrete them. As both free radicals and the toxins that help create them contribute to the onset of cancer, garlic is one of the most potent aids to health that you can find.

Cleansing and toning

The cleansing powers of garlic are formidable. It is an age-old remedy for parasites in the stomach and intestines. It is excellent for clearing respiratory ailments (onions are good, too) and is a decongestant, making it very helpful in cases of catarrh, bronchitis and asthma. It is also an unusually effective cleanser and toner of the liver.

Garlic is also renowned for its beneficial effects on the heart and the circulation. It can reduce high blood pressure – it contains a substance called allicin, which dilates the blood vessels and reduces clotting – and it can lower cholesterol levels. It thins the blood and this helps improve the sluggish circulation that results in cold hands and feet, and also counters diseases of the arteries. Allicin is excreted through the lungs, bowels, skin and urinary system and in the process detoxifies all of them.

Garlic contains sulphur, which helps cleanse the liver and is also believed to inhibit the growth of tumours. Onion can reduce blood sugar, which explains its use in the folk remedy for diabetes.

Choosing, storing and using

Choose firm bulbs with a papery top layer and no sprouts. Keep in a cool, dry place or the refrigerator and use as soon as possible after purchase.

There are numerous ways of eating garlic and onions. Most commonly, they are quickly fried for use in all kinds of recipes, though they can be used raw in salads or dressings and even be made into a juice, but only in very small quantities and mixed with other ingredients. They can also be roasted in the oven and served as a side dish.

The Benefits
- Fights colds and viral infections
- Acts as a natural antibiotic
- Helps improve circulation
- Reduces cholesterol
- Tones and cleanses the liver
- Expels parasites
- Strengthens immune system
- Reduces high blood pressure

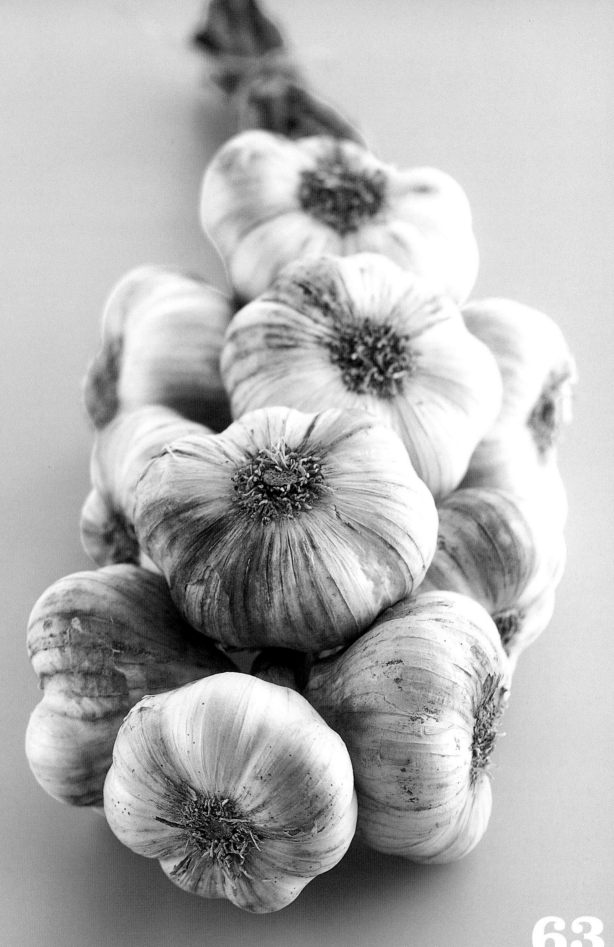

chicken with forty garlic cloves

This is a classic French recipe which uses an enormous amount of garlic. It will perfume the house as it cooks and the garlic will become milder in flavour and much sweeter.

Preparation time: 15 minutes
Cooking time: 1 hour 50 minutes
Serves 6

2 kg (4 lb) oven-ready chicken, giblets removed
2 tablespoons olive oil
40 whole garlic cloves, unpeeled
8 shallots
150 ml (¼ pint) dry white wine
150 ml (¼ pint) chicken stock
4 thyme sprigs
1 lemon, halved
500 g (1 lb) small carrots
sea salt and pepper

1 Pat the chicken dry and season inside and out with salt and pepper. Heat the oil in a large flameproof casserole and brown the chicken on all sides.

2 Remove the chicken and add the garlic and shallots to the casserole in one layer. Sauté gently for about 5-7 minutes, shaking the pan frequently. Slowly pour the wine and stock into the pan. Return the chicken to the casserole and sprinkle with the thyme and salt. Add the halved lemon and cover the casserole tightly.

3 Cook in a preheated oven, 190°C (375°F), Gas Mark 5, for 1 hour, then add the carrots and cook for a further 30 minutes. Remove the lid and put the casserole back in the oven for a final 10-15 minutes to crisp the chicken skin.

4 Carve the chicken and serve with the pan juices and the creamy garlic cloves and roasted carrots. (Diners peel the garlic cloves as they eat.)

garlic & almond soup

Preparation time: 15 minutes,
    plus soaking and chilling
Serves 6

50 g (2 oz) bread
125 g (4 oz) raisins
125 g (4 oz) blanched
    almonds, toasted
3 tablespoons olive oil
3 garlic cloves, crushed or
    roughly chopped
900 ml (1½ pints) milk or water
hyssop or borage flowers,
    to serve

This soup is quite rich and should be served in small quantities. It was known in ancient Rome and has always been considered highly beneficial to good health, with its antibacterial and heart-protecting properties.

1 Tear the bread into small rough pieces and put them and the raisins in separate bowls and cover each with water. Leave to soak for 30-60 minutes or until the raisins are plump.

2 Remove the bread from the water and squeeze dry to remove the excess moisture. Put the bread in a food processor or blender with the almonds and blend to a smooth paste, or use a pestle and mortar.

3 Add the olive oil, garlic, raisins and milk or water and blend once again to make a smooth soup.

4 Chill the soup thoroughly in the refrigerator for 2-3 hours to allow the flavours to mingle. Serve in small bowls topped with hyssop or borage flowers.

honey

Honey is not only deliciously sweet – twice as sweet as sugar, in fact – it also possesses a range of health-giving properties. It is a potent antiseptic and a well-known remedy for colds, coughs and sore throats. However, it should be used in moderation as it is high in calories and, like sugar itself, can cause tooth decay.

An antiseptic – internal and external

As an antiseptic, honey is renowned for calming coughs and fevers. One of the most common surviving folk remedies is a drink made with hot water, honey and lemon for treating colds and other respiratory ailments. Honey also helps relieve coughs, catarrh and sinus problems. Its antiseptic and antibacterial properties protect against numerous infectious diseases that affect the digestive tract. It is an excellent natural remedy for all kinds of gastroenteritis, including travellers' tummy bugs – and is even recommended for this purpose by the World Health Organization. Half a teaspoon of honey daily helps to soothe peptic ulcers.

Hay fever

Rather unexpectedly, perhaps, honey can help with hay fever – an allergic respiratory reaction often triggered by pollen. Naturopaths believe that taking a teaspoon of honey containing some of the wax from the honeycomb cells every day will build up your resistance. It is important, though, to buy honey that has been produced locally and which is natural, unprocessed and organic.

A convalescent food

Honey is a perfect food for convalescence, being easily eaten and digested, and full of energizing sugars, and also because it stimulates production of serotonin, which has a relaxing and mood-enhancing effect. It also contains a wealth of minerals, as well as vitamin C and numerous B vitamins. Its healing properties are believed to speed up recovery in some widely varied conditions, including liver and kidney ailments, circulation problems and arthritis.

Bee products

It isn't just honey that comes out of the hive. Other bee products include propolis, royal jelly and pollen. Propolis is an even stronger antibiotic than honey, while royal jelly has been found to have some quite astonishing results – lowering blood pressure, speeding up the healing process, reducing cholesterol, stimulating the immune system and increasing energy. Royal jelly contains all the B vitamins, as well as vitamin C and all of the essential amino acids, which are responsible for the growth, repair and regeneration of cells.

Choosing, storing and using

Look for cold-pressed honey and buy it, if possible, direct from the farm. Most honey you will find in the supermarket goes through a heating process that filters out some of the most nutritious elements. Buying unfiltered honey is particularly important for hay fever sufferers, as this helps desensitize them to the effects of pollen.

Store honey in the kitchen cupboard – its antimicrobial properties mean it doesn't go off. It is twice as sweet as sugar so you need less of it when using it as a sweetener. However, remember that heat reduces its antibiotic properties so add it to cooked dishes later than you would sugar.

The Benefits
- Fights bacteria
- Provides energy
- Protects immune system
- Soothes coughs, colds, respiratory infections
- Relieves stomach upsets
- Reduces hay fever symptoms

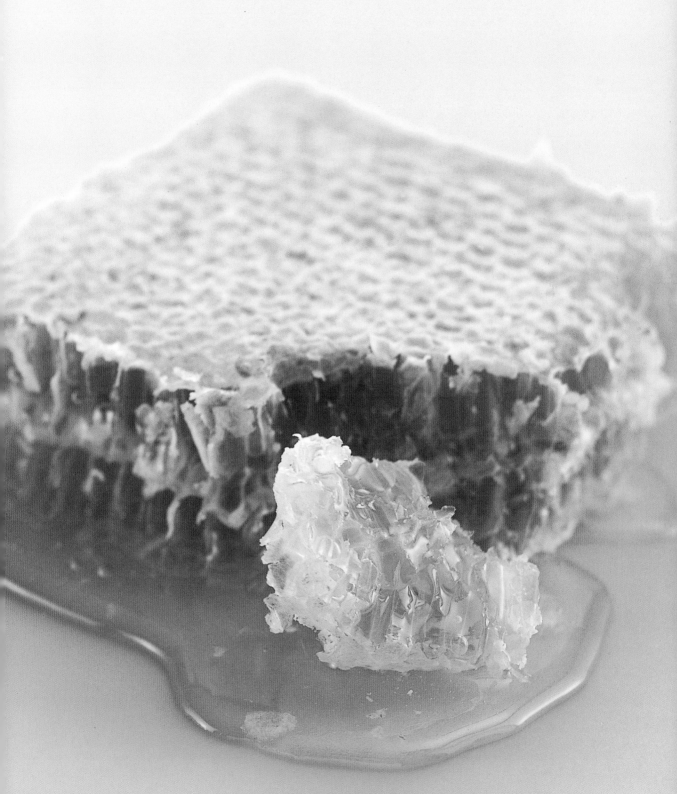

67

honey & ginger yogurt ice

Preparation time: 15 minutes,
    plus freezing
Cooking time: 10 minutes
Serves 4–6

7.5 cm (3 inch) piece of fresh root
    ginger
8 tablespoons thick honey
6 tablespoons water
600 ml (1 pint) thick yogurt

To serve:
slices of fresh mango, pineapple
    or lychees
extra honey, for drizzling
    (optional)

Honey and yogurt frozen with ginger makes a light and refreshing ice to serve with fresh fruit. Increase or decrease the honey according to personal taste and, if you prefer, leave out the ginger or use chopped stem ginger instead.

1 Peel the ginger, finely chop the flesh and place it in a small saucepan with 2 tablespoons of the honey and the water and bring slowly to the boil. Reduce the heat, cover the pan and simmer gently for 10 minutes. Remove from the heat and leave to cool.

2 When the ginger and honey mixture is cold, stir it mixture into the thick yogurt with the remaining honey and pour into a chilled freezer container. Cover the container and freeze for 3-4 hours.

3 Using a chilled fork, stir the yogurt mixture to break up the ice crystals. Return to the freezer and repeat this mixing and freezing process twice more, then leave the yogurt ice to freeze until firm.

4 Remove the yogurt ice from the freezer 20 minutes before serving. Scoop into small bowls and serve with slices of fresh mango, pineapple or lychees. If you like, drizzle the top of the yogurt ice with extra honey.

honey & yogurt with prune purée

This can be served for breakfast, as a snack or as a pudding. Leave the layers intact or gently mix them all together, as you prefer. Add extra honey if you like.

Preparation time: 10 minutes
Cooking time: 8 minutes
Serves 4

250 g (8 oz) ready-to-eat
   pitted prunes
juice and finely grated rind of
   1 lemon
8–12 tablespoons clear honey
450 ml (¾ pint) thick
   natural yogurt
1–2 tablespoons crunchy muesli

1 Put the prunes into a saucepan with the lemon juice, grated rind and 8 tablespoons cold water. Cover and simmer very gently for 6-8 minutes. Remove the pan from the heat and tip the mixture into a food processor or blender and blend to a coarse purée.

2 Divide the prune purée between 4 glasses and cover each with a thick layer of honey, then add a layer of thick yogurt and sprinkle the top with crunchy muesli. Serve immediately.

Preparation time: 10 minutes
Cooking time: 4 minutes
Serves 4

4 thick slices of German fruit
   bread
4 tablespoons mascarpone
6-8 tablespoons thick honeycomb
finely grated rind of
   ½ small lemon
75 g (3 oz) blueberries
   and raspberries
½ teaspoon grated nutmeg
fruit juice, to serve

Nothing can be better than lashings of honey on warm toast. This glamorous version of our breakfast staple can be served at any time of the day and makes an excellent pudding. The mascarpone could quite easily be replaced with a small scoop of the best vanilla ice cream or, for those watching calories, low-fat cream cheese or thick natural yogurt would be just as good.

1 Toast the bread until golden brown and firm. Beat the mascarpone with 2 teaspoons of the honey and the finely grated lemon rind.

2 Put a little of the remaining honey on the warm toast, then place a spoonful of the lemon mascarpone on top and spread it over the toast.

3 Scatter a few berries over and around the toast and drizzle the remaining honey over it. Grate the nutmeg over the warm toast. Serve with a knife and fork and a large glass of fruit juice.

honey & mascarpone breakfast bread with berries

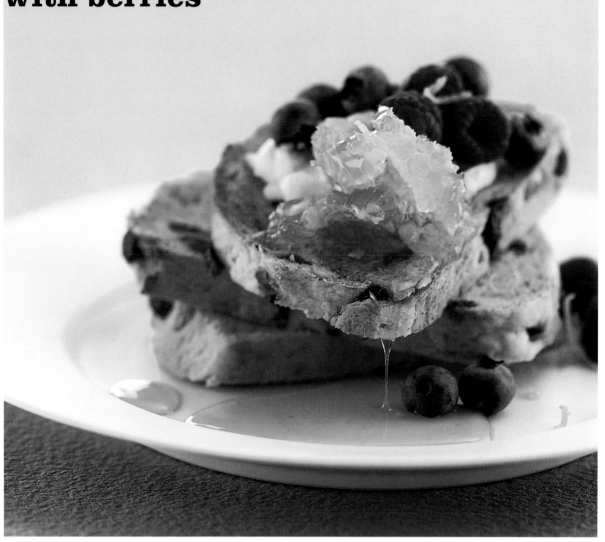

The World Health Organization recommends honey as an excellent natural remedy for all kinds of gastroenteritis.

mangoes & papayas

These delicious tropical fruits, are full of powerful antioxidants and are potent detoxifiers of the entire system. They are highly beneficial for the digestive system too, and for skin and nails.

Beta-carotene

Like all orange and yellow fruits and vegetables, mangoes and papayas contain beta-carotene. The darker the colour of a fruit, the more beta-carotene it contains so papayas have particularly high levels. The body converts the beta-carotene to vitamin A and, as these fruits have plenty of vitamin C as well, this makes them powerful antioxidants. Mangoes also contain vitamin E – the third antioxidant vitamin – and both fruits contain iron and zinc. This high level of antioxidants puts them at the forefront of immune health protection, safeguarding against all kinds of risks, from passing infections to cancer.

Strength and beauty

Mangoes and papayas have a deeply detoxifying effect on the body which shows visibly by improving skin texture, fighting off wrinkles and giving the complexion a bloom. They also strengthen the nails. They are an energizing fruit, too, and make a nutritious snack whenever your energy level dips.

Digestive aids

Papayas are renowned as an aid to digestion. They contain the enzyme papain, which digests protein, and they cleanse and soothe the digestive tract, reducing inflammation and intestinal infection and problems such as constipation and flatulence. They also get rid of intestinal parasites. Mangoes are also soothing to the digestive system, and especially beneficial for problems like indigestion. They are particularly powerful cleansers of the blood and the kidneys, which further detoxifies the body.

Choosing, storing and using

Mangoes and papayas should be eaten ripe, when their flavour and nutrition levels are at their best. The papaya skin should be yellow and green, and should be firm but not hard to the touch. If the papaya has a strong fragrance, you know it's ready to eat. Ripe mangoes should have a red rather than a yellow skin, and, like the papaya, should be firm to the touch. Store mangoes and papayas in the refrigerator, or leave them in the fruit bowl to ripen. Great care must be taken when handling papayas because the skin and the seeds can cause itching for some people. Always wash your hands after touching papayas, and never touch your eyes until you have done so, as this can cause stinging. To eat, cut in half, scoop out the seeds and eat the flesh. Mangoes and papayas also make wonderful juice if you have a juicer in the kitchen, though the juice is too thick to drink alone and should be mixed with a more watery fruit, such as apple.

The Benefits
- Powerful antioxidant
- Boost the immune system
- Anti-cancer
- Improve skin and nails
- Soothe digestive system
- Provide energy

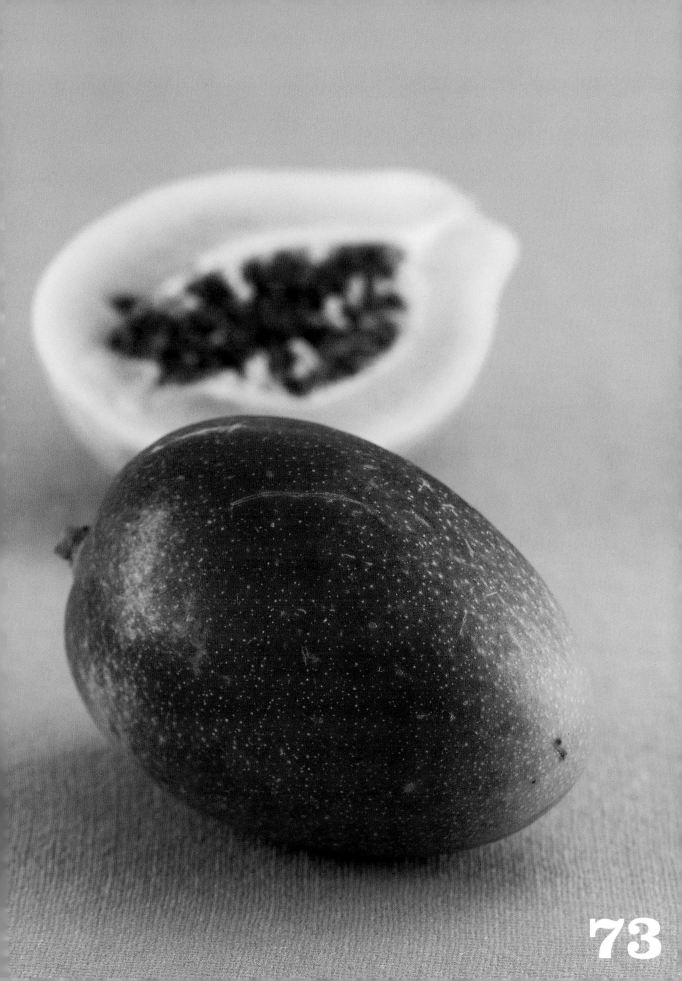

papaya & lime salad

Papaya and lime complement each other wonderfully and boost the vitamin C intake. This simple, but utterly delicious fruit salad can be served for breakfast with muesli and yogurt, as a pudding with crème fraîche or on its own.

Preparation time: 15 minutes
Cooking time: 4 minutes
Serves 4

3 firm ripe papayas
2 limes
2 teaspoons golden caster sugar
75 g (3 oz) blanched
**   almonds, toasted**

1 Cut the papayas in half, scoop out the seeds and discard. Peel the halves, cut the flesh roughly into dice and place in a bowl.

2 Finely grate the rind of both limes, then squeeze 1 of the limes and reserve the juice. Cut the pith off the second lime and segment the flesh over the bowl of diced papaya to catch the juice. Add the lime segments and grated lime rind to the papaya.

3 Put the lime juice into a small saucepan with the sugar and heat gently until the sugar has dissolved. Remove from the heat and allow to cool.

4 When the sweetened lime juice has cooled, pour it over the fruit and toss thoroughly. Add the toasted almonds to the fruit salad and serve.

oriental papaya & mango salad

Fresh salads of fruit and vegetables are popular in the Far East. This version of the Thai *som tam* is light and fruity and delicious served with grilled fish, meats or satay and rice. It is important to use fruits that are still slightly unripe and firm as they are easier to prepare and not too sweet.

Preparation time: 20 minutes
Serves 4

1 small, firm papaya
1 small, firm mango
3 tomatoes
1 garlic clove, roughly chopped
1 red onion, finely chopped
1 small red chilli, roughly
  chopped (optional)
2 tablespoons roughly chopped
  roasted peanuts or pine nuts
2 tablespoons chopped coriander
  leaves
2 tablespoons Thai fish sauce
2 teaspoons light brown
  muscovado sugar
3 tablespoons lime or lemon
  juice

To serve:
grilled meat or fish
boiled red rice

1 Cut the papayas in half, scoop out the seeds and discard. Cut the mango into two pieces either side of the stone. Peel away the skin and discard it. Roughly grate the fruits or thinly slice them into fine strips.

2 Quarter the tomatoes and put them into a large mortar or bowl with the garlic, red onion and chilli, if using, and lightly pound with a pestle or the end of a rolling pin for 1-2 minutes or until they are well mixed and the tomatoes are mashed.

3 Add the papaya and mango and pound lightly to mix. Add the peanuts or pine nuts, coriander, fish sauce, sugar and lime or lemon juice and pound again to mix thoroughly.

4 Spoon the mixture into a small bowl and serve with grilled meat or fish and boiled red rice.

Preparation time: 15 minutes,
    plus marinating
Cooking time: 6 minutes
Serves 4

4 x 150 g (5 oz) swordfish steaks
4 tablespoons olive oil
1 tablespoon chopped parsley
1 teaspoon thyme leaves
1 garlic clove, crushed
finely grated rind of 1 lime
sea salt and pepper

Raw mango chutney:
1 large, firm, ripe mango
½ small red onion
1 small red pepper, deseeded
1 spring onion, finely shredded
1 tablespoon chopped flat
    leaf parsley
3 tablespoons lime juice
2 tablespoons extra virgin
    olive oil
baby spinach leaves, to serve
thick lime wedges, to garnish

Mangoes are excellent for the digestive system and a good natural detoxifier. Here they are perfectly balanced by the flavour of lime and used, uncooked, as an accompaniment to grilled or griddled fish.

1 Put the swordfish steaks into a shallow bowl. Mix together the olive oil, parsley, thyme, crushed garlic, finely grated lime rind and salt and pepper. Pour over the swordfish and leave to marinate for 30-60 minutes.

2 Meanwhile, to make the raw mango chutney, cut the mango in half, discard the stone and peel off the skin. Finely dice the mango flesh and put it into a bowl. Very finely chop the red onion and red pepper and add to the mango.

3 Add the shredded spring onion, parsley, lime juice and olive oil to the bowl and carefully mix together. Cover and leave at room temperature for 1 hour to allow the flavours to infuse.

4 Heat a grill or griddle and cook the swordfish for 2-3 minutes on each side, depending on the thickness of the fish. Put a pile of raw baby spinach leaves on each plate, place the hot swordfish steaks on top and spoon the mango chutney over and around them. Serve immediately and garnish with thick wedges of lime.

raw mango chutney with swordfish

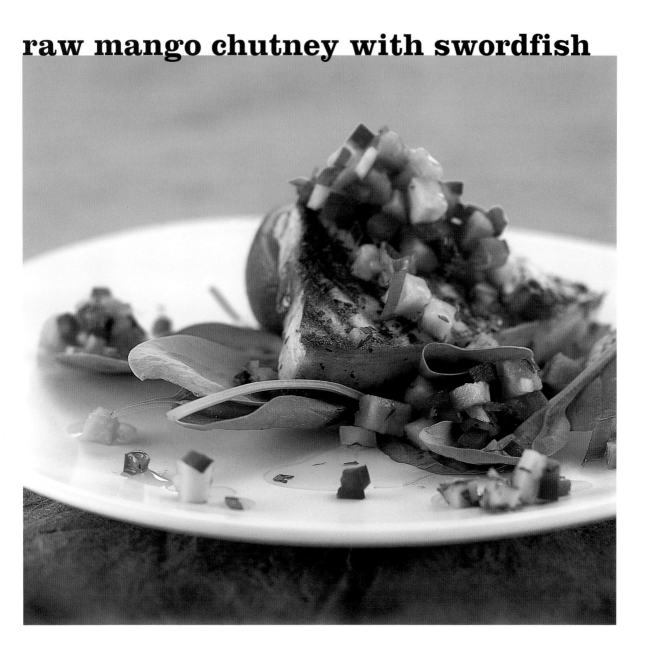

Mangoes and papayas have a deeply detoxifying effect on the body which shows visibly by reducing wrinkles, improving skin texture and giving the complexion a bloom.

nuts

Like honey, nuts tend to be high in calories, but their health-giving properties mean they are too good to miss out of your diet. Their protein content makes them vital for strict vegetarians who do not eat meat, fish or dairy products. Cashews, walnuts, pine nuts, hazelnuts, almonds - and coconuts - are among the most nutritious.

Heart health

Many nuts, notably almonds, walnuts, hazelnuts and coconuts, have high levels of vitamin E, which protects against heart disease. Although most nuts are high in fat, this is mainly, except in the case of coconuts, monounsaturated fat, so most nuts do contribute to lowering cholesterol, if eaten in moderation. Walnuts contain linoleic acid which not only lowers cholesterol, it also reduces blood pressure and helps prevent blood clotting. Some nuts also help to build red blood cells and prevent anaemia.

Antioxidants

Besides the antioxidant vitamin E, many nuts contain vitamin C - in particular, Brazil nuts, chestnuts, hazelnuts and coconuts - while hazelnuts, chestnuts and cashews contain beta-carotene, which the body turns into vitamin A. These antioxidant vitamins are, of course, essential to immune health and build up resistance to disease. Of the antioxidant minerals, Brazil nuts and walnuts contain selenium, while almonds, pine nuts and hazelnuts have zinc. Many nuts also contain a wide range of B vitamins, responsible for metabolizing food into energy and strengthening the nervous system.

Strengthening powers

High in both protein and carbohydrates, nuts are an energizing food, useful for anyone who is underweight or convalescing. They are a good source of protein for strict vegetarians and people with small appetites. The high levels of calcium in walnuts, almonds and cashew nuts strengthen bones, hair and teeth.

Many nuts are anti-inflammatory, too. This helps to reduce the symptoms of rheumatoid arthritis and inflammatory skin conditions, such as rashes. Coconuts have high levels of folic acid, which protects against spina bifida in the unborn child, and phytoestrogens (see page 30), which are helpful for women who suffer from PMS or menopausal side effects.

Choosing, storing and using

Buy nuts in their raw form and as unprocessed as possible, that is without any added salt, or blanched, flaked or ground. You can shell nuts and eat them as they are, or roast them gently, which often releases more of their flavour. You can use them in a wide variety of sweet and savoury recipes or turn them into dips or spreads.

The exception to all this is the coconut. This is actually a fruit, not a nut, and it comes in various forms, depending on its age. The youngest is the green coconut, which is full of highly nutritious, fizzy coconut milk or water - and this you drink with a straw. At the other extreme, the coconut meat can be dried to make copra. Coconut is available in many forms - dried, fresh and canned. Always buy the freshest and least processed version you can find.

Nut oils are excellent for salad dressings, but use only the cold-pressed varieties. Store in a cool, dark place.

The Benefits
- Protect against heart disease
- Lower high cholesterol
- Strengthen bones, teeth, hair
- Alleviate symptoms of PMS and menopause
- Provide energy
- Strengthen blood and prevent anaemia

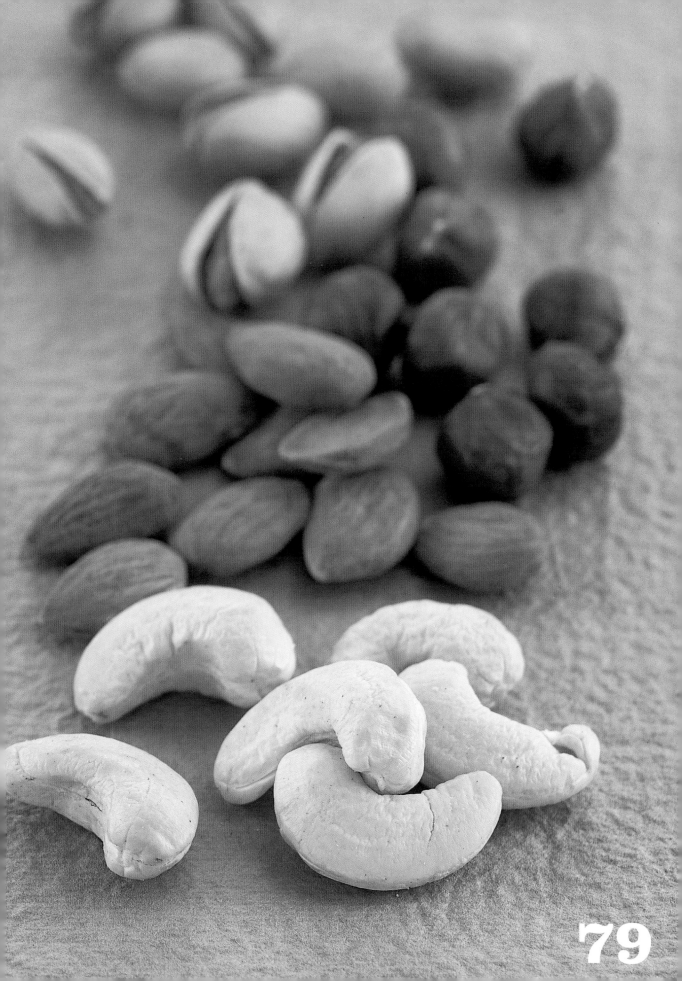

pan-fried monkfish
with toasted hazelnut oil

Nuts can be added with breadcrumbs to fish and meat as a protective crust or stirred into the pan at the end of cooking. Here hazelnuts are lightly toasted to increase their flavour then added to the olive oil and used to dress pan-fried fish. Use pine nuts, cashews or walnuts, if you prefer.

Preparation time: 20 minutes
Cooking time: 15 minutes
Serves 4

75 g (3 oz) hazelnuts or almonds,
  roughly chopped
250 g (8 oz) green beans,
  trimmed
750 g (1 ½ lb) monkfish or sea
  bass
8 tablespoons olive oil
2–3 tablespoons lemon juice
2 tablespoons chopped flat leaf
  parsley
sea salt and pepper

1 Toast the hazelnut or almonds in a large dry frying pan, shaking the pan frequently to prevent them burning. Remove the nuts from the pan and cool slightly.

2 Bring a pan of water to the boil, plunge the green beans into the water and cook for 1 minute. Drain well and refresh under running cold water.

3 Remove and discard any skin from the fish and cut the fish into thick pieces. Season well with salt and pepper.

4 Heat 3 tablespoons oil in a large frying pan until hot. Add half the fish pieces to the pan; do not overcrowd the pan or the heat of the pan will reduce. Sauté the fish on both sides for 2-3 minutes or until cooked through and tinged with brown. Remove from the pan and add the remaining pieces of fish and cook as before.

5 Remove the second batch of fish and add the remaining oil to the pan with the chopped nuts and heat gently to warm the nuts through. Return all the fish pieces to the pan and carefully toss the fish with the nuts.

6 Add the lemon juice, chopped parsley and salt and pepper. Remove the pan from the heat and serve the fish on individual plates on a bed of green beans with the nut and parsley oil poured over the top.

walnut pesto genoese with green beans

Preparation time: 10 minutes
Cooking time: 22 minutes
Serves 4

3 garlic cloves, crushed
150 ml (¼ pint) extra virgin
    olive oil
50 g (2 oz) basil leaves
50 g (2 oz) walnuts,
    roughly chopped
1 tablespoon freshly grated
    Parmesan cheese
pinch of dried chilli flakes
175 g (6 oz) small waxy
    potatoes, unpeeled
400 g (13 oz) fusilli or
    orecchetti pasta
125 g (4 oz) green beans,
    trimmed and halved
sea salt and pepper

To serve:
50 g (2 oz) walnut halves,
    roughly chopped
extra virgin olive oil (optional)
Parmesan shavings

Pasta with waxy potatoes, green beans and pesto is a traditional recipe from Liguria in Italy, the region around Genoa, but in this version walnuts have been used and add a slightly bitter taste. Brazils, the more usual pine nuts, sunflower seeds or pumpkin seeds can all be used in their place.

1 Put the crushed garlic in a food processor or blender with the olive oil and basil leaves and blend to a rough paste, or use a pestle or mortar. Add the roughly chopped walnuts, salt, pepper, Parmesan cheese and chilli flakes and blend to a textured paste.

2 Halve or quarter the potatoes if large. Add to a pan of boiling water and boil for 8-10 minutes or until just cooked, but still firm. Cook the pasta in plenty of boiling water for 10-12 minutes or until just al dente. In a separate pan boil the green beans for 4-5 minutes.

3 Drain the potatoes, pasta and beans and return all three to one large pan. Add the pesto sauce and toss together while still hot. Add the extra roughly chopped walnuts to the top of the pasta and serve immediately with extra olive oil, if liked, and shavings of Parmesan cheese.

A light, warm salad cooked in groundnut oil and finished with toasted nuts. You could use almonds or hazelnuts instead of the toasted peanuts, if you prefer.

Preparation time: 25 minutes, plus soaking
Cooking time: 10 minutes
Serves 4

175 g (6 oz) thin rice noodles
500 g (1 lb) baby squid, skinned, cleaned and gutted
3 red chillies, deseeded and finely chopped
3 garlic cloves, crushed
2 tablespoons chopped coriander
3 tablespoons groundnut oil
175 g (6 oz) peanuts
125 g (4 oz) green beans, shredded
3 tablespoons Thai fish sauce
1 teaspoon caster sugar
3 tablespoons lemon juice
handful of coriander leaves
thick lime wedges, to serve

1 Fill a large pan or bowl with boiling water, add the noodles and leave to soak for 5-8 minutes or until they are soft. Drain well and rinse in cold water.

2 Cut the squid bodies in half lengthways and make a series of slashes in a diagonal criss-cross pattern on the underside of each piece of squid.

3 Mix together the chopped red chillies, garlic and coriander. Toss through the squid pieces, then leave to stand for 20 minutes.

4 Heat the oil in a wok or large frying pan and toast the peanuts for 2-3 minutes until golden brown. Remove from the oil and reserve. Do not overcook them as they will continue to cook once out of the pan. Add the squid to the oil and quickly stir-fry for 2-3 minutes or until the squid pieces have begun to curl and the flesh turns white. Remove from the pan and reserve with the peanuts.

5 Add the shredded beans and stir-fry for 2 minutes. Mix the fish sauce, caster sugar and lemon juice with 3 tablespoons water, add to the pan and cook for a further 1 minute. Remove the pan from the heat, add the drained noodles and toss together well. Add the toasted peanuts, cooked squid and coriander leaves, and toss again. Eat while warm or leave to cool. Serve with thick lime wedges.

peanut & squid salad
with rice noodles

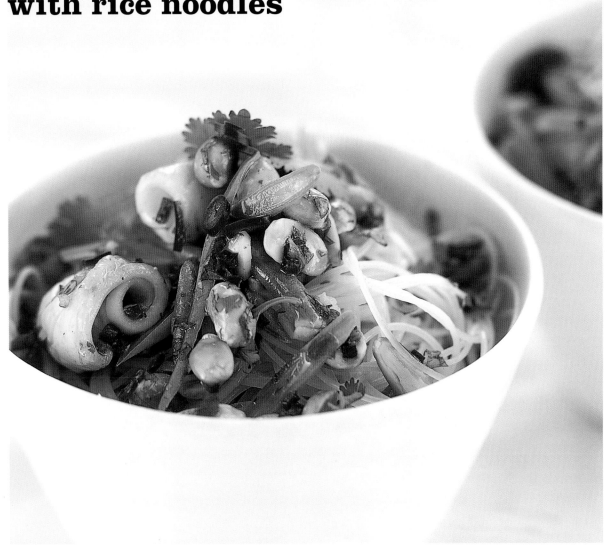

High in both protein and carbohydrates, nuts are an energizing food, useful for anyone who is underweight or convalescing.

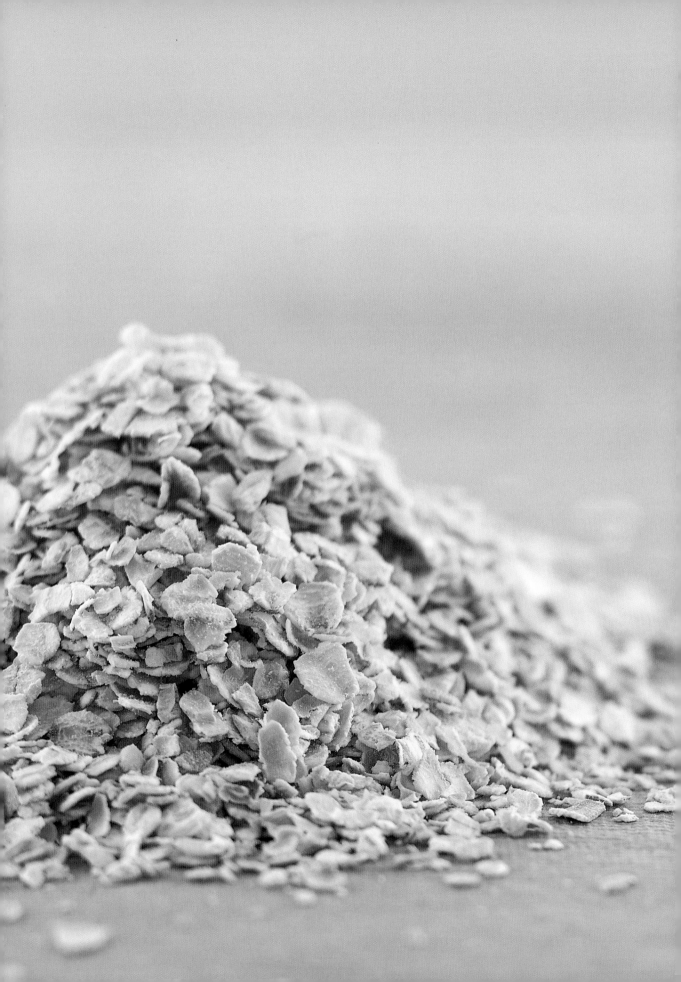

oats

One of the most nutritious grains, oats can often be tolerated by the growing numbers of people who have an allergy to wheat. Oatmeal and rolled oats do not go through any refining processes, so they are whole foods, losing none of their nutritional properties.

Body building

Oats are full of protein and minerals and are helpful for building strong bones, teeth and connective tissue and for boosting energy generally. They also contain high levels of calcium and phosphorus. They are easily digested and so are traditionally regarded as a good food for convalescence, particularly after childbirth, as they are also believed to tone the uterus. They are renowned for helping to strengthen the nervous system and for their tranquillizing and relaxing effects. Studies have shown that these effects extend even to people suffering from withdrawal symptoms after long use of cigarettes, tranquillizers and antidepressant drugs. A folk remedy for insomnia advises sleeping on a pillow or mattress filled with oats.

The digestive connection

Oats contain a soluble fibre that acts on the digestive system in several ways. They provide dietary bulk, which improves the digestive process and prevents constipation or eases it if the condition already exists. Oats are a soothing food for the digestive tract too, notably for conditions such as gastritis and irritable bowel syndrome. And, because they sweep food – and carcinogens – through the gut they may also help prevent bowel cancer. Oats reduce the absorption of carbohydrates into the blood stream, stabilizing blood sugar levels which, in turn, may help diabetics, and also reduces mood swings. This is particularly useful when mood swings are one of the symptoms of premenstrual syndrome (PMS), as oats may also stabilize oestrogen levels and reduce water retention.

Soluble fibre

One of the most significant benefits of oats is in helping to maintain cardiovascular health. Their soluble fibre helps to lower cholesterol and generally boost cardiovascular health, lowering high blood pressure. Oats also contain high levels of iron, which is essential for the formation of healthy red blood cells and their function in taking oxygen around the body, as well as for preventing iron-deficiency anaemia, notably in women who suffer from very heavy or prolonged menstrual periods.

Oats are also believed to stimulate the thyroid gland, which makes the hormones that regulate the body's metabolizing of food into energy.

Choosing, storing and using

Choose rolled oats and oatmeal rather than any of the instant varieties for making porridge. Store in a dark, cool place, preferably in an airtight jar, and use as soon as possible, but certainly within three months of purchase.

Oats can be eaten raw or cooked, the best-known cooked recipe being porridge. They can be soaked in fruit juice and eaten raw with added fruit as a nutritious cereal and used as a thickening agent in a wide variety of cooked recipes.

The Benefits
- Reduce cholesterol
- Stabilize blood sugar levels
- Soothing and tranquillizing
- Build strong bones and teeth
- Stimulate thyroid gland
- Prevent constipation

oated herrings with raw artichoke salad

Oatmeal makes a healthy crust for fish and cooks to a crisp crumb. Here the herrings are served with a classic Italian raw artichoke salad. The small baby artichokes are the best ones to use, but if you cannot find them, use two thinly sliced bulbs and coat them in the same lemon and mustard dressing.

Preparation time: 25 minutes
Cooking time: 25 minutes
Serves 4

4 large or 8 small
  herrings, gutted
125 g (4 oz) pinhead oatmeal
7 tablespoons olive oil
2 teaspoons Dijon mustard
juice of 3 lemons
8 baby globe artichokes
2 teaspoons wholegrain mustard
salt and pepper
lemon wedges, to serve

1 Place the herrings on a board and slit open the stomachs, pressing gently along the backbone until the herrings lie flat.

2 Season the oatmeal with plenty of pepper and a small pinch of salt. Mix 3 tablespoons of the olive oil with the Dijon mustard. Brush the mixture over one side of each herring in turn, then lay them in the oatmeal and flip over and coat the second side. Do this with all the herrings, then put them in a roasting tin.

3 Bake the herrings in a preheated oven, 200°C (400°F), Gas Mark 6, for 20-25 minutes or until the fish have just cooked through and the oatmeal crust is beginning to turn golden brown.

4 Meanwhile, fill a bowl with water and add the juice of 1 of the lemons to the water with the lemon shells. Have this lemon water ready before you start to prepare the artichokes, as the artichokes will turn brown when exposed to the air.

5 Take an artichoke and cut off the stalk end. Remove the outside leaves until just the tender inside leaves remain. Cut off the tips of these leaves and immediately plunge the prepared artichoke into the lemon water. Repeat with the remaining artichokes.

6 To make the dressing, mix the remaining olive oil with the remaining lemon juice, wholegrain mustard and salt and pepper. Working with one artichoke at a time, lift it out of the water, cut it in half and remove the hairy choke with a teaspoon. Slice the artichoke thinly and put the slices into a bowl. Pour the lemon and mustard dressing over the slices of artichoke and toss well. Repeat with the remaining artichokes.

7 When the fish are cooked through, arrange them on a bed of artichoke salad with wedges of lemon and serve immediately.

strawberry & apricot oat crumble

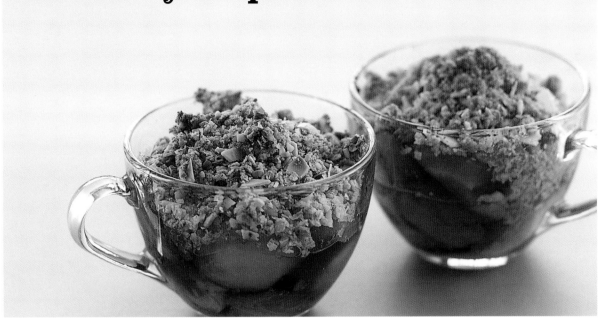

Preparation time: 20 minutes
Cooking time: 30 minutes
Serves 4–6

250 g (8 oz) strawberries
500 g (1 lb) apricots
finely grated rind of ½ lemon
1 tablespoon lemon juice
1 vanilla pod, split lengthways
2 tablespoons clear honey or soft
  dark brown sugar
125 g (4 oz) medium rolled oats
75 g (3 oz) wholemeal flour
75 g (3 oz) butter
50 g (2 oz) almonds or Brazil
  nuts, toasted and
  finely chopped
1 tablespoon soft light
  brown sugar
fromage frais, thick natural
  yogurt or crème fraîche,
  to serve

Rolled oats make a fine crumble topping, and here they are combined with finely chopped nuts for extra texture. Any fruit from apple to peach and blackberry to blueberry can be used in place of the strawberries and apricots.

1 Hull the strawberries and halve any large ones. Cut the apricots in half, remove the stones and roughly quarter the fruit.

2 Mix the apricots and strawberries with the grated lemon rind and lemon juice and pack into a 625-750 g (1¼-1½ lb) ovenproof dish. Put the halved vanilla pod into the middle of the dish and drizzle the honey over the fruit or sprinkle over the dark brown sugar.

3 Mix the rolled oats with the wholemeal flour and then rub the butter into the mixture until it becomes a rough crumble. Add the chopped nuts and light brown sugar and mix well.

4 Spoon the mixture over the prepared fruit and bake in a preheated oven, 180°C (350°F), Gas Mark 4, for 25-30 minutes or until the crumble topping is golden brown and crisp. Serve with fromage frais, yogurt or crème fraîche. Don't forget to discard the vanilla pod before serving.

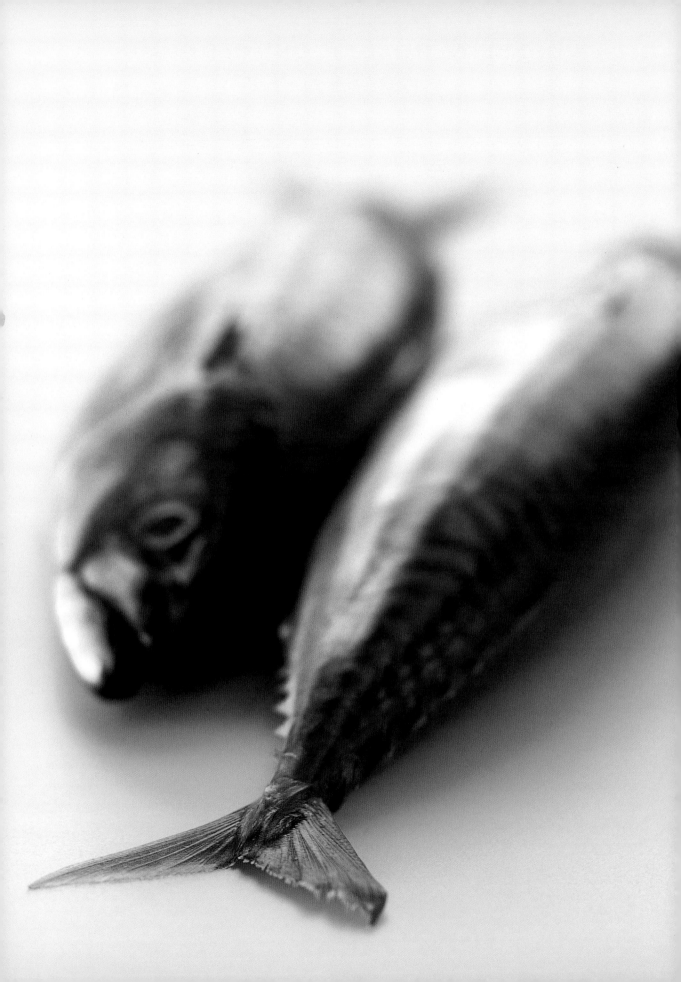

oily fish

There are several kinds of highly nutritious oily fish. These include salmon, whitebait, tuna, mackerel, herring and sardines - all of which contain the highly protective Omega-3 fatty acids.

The essential fatty acids

All oily fish contain Omega-3 essential fatty acids. They are called essential because they cannot be made within the body, but must be obtained from food. These fish oils provide a range of health benefits. They improve memory and other brain functions - so fish really is 'brain food' - protect the heart against disease, prevent blood clots and strengthen cardiovascular health. They also protect against some of the risk factors that lead to heart disease, lowering both cholesterol levels and high blood pressure. Essential fatty acids reduce the risk of stroke, too.

Omega-3 fatty acids help in a wide range of other conditions. There is evidence that they improve rheumatoid arthritis, both reducing the swelling of joints and making them less painful. They may also reduce the symptoms of premenstrual syndrome (PMS), especially mood swings and irritability. They also have a beneficial effect on various inflammatory skin conditions, including psoriasis, dermatitis and eczema, as well as improving dry skin generally. Omega-3 essential fatty acids may also help to reduce cellulite.

The cancer-fighting mineral

Fish is one of the best sources of the mineral selenium. This is one of the antioxidants that protect against the development of cancer. It does this by detoxifying the body, attacking free radicals (see page 8) and removing heavy metals, such as mercury, from the system. Selenium also strengthens the immune system generally, improving resistance to infection and raising the white blood cell count. Oily fish gives a double dose of heart health, as both its essential fatty acids and selenium protect against heart disease.

Antioxidant E

Many kinds of oily fish contain another important antioxidant - vitamin E - which works in tandem with selenium to protect the heart. Vitamin C also enhances the benefits of both these antioxidants, so eating fish with green, leafy vegetables makes a potent health package.

Tuna benefits

Fresh tuna is particularly good for rheumatoid arthritis. It contains not only the Omega-3 fatty acids that benefit the complaint, but also biotin and vitamin B3, which are anti-inflammatory and so further reduce the painful symptoms of rheumatoid arthritis. Tuna also contains tryptophan, an amino acid that helps regulate sleep.

Choosing, storing and using

Not surprisingly, fresh is best when it comes to fish. Freshness shows in firm flesh and a clear eye, not a dull or opaque one. If buying farmed salmon, check it is not genetically modified (GM). Keep fish in the refrigerator and eat on the day of purchase.

Fish can be eaten raw, smoked or cooked in any number of ways - though methods involving batter and frying should be avoided. It cooks very quickly when baked or grilled.

The Benefits
- **Strengthen immune system**
- **Protect against heart disease**
- **Protect against cancer**
- **Reduce rheumatoid arthritis symptoms**
- **Improve inflammatory skin conditions**
- **Improve dry skin**
- **Lower cholesterol and blood pressure**

smoked mackerel
on toast with rocket

Preparation time: 15 minutes
Cooking time: 10 minutes
Serves 4

1 garlic clove, crushed
2 tablespoons pine nuts
4 tablespoons roughly chopped
   flat leaf parsley
1 tablespoon lemon juice
6 tablespoons olive oil
4 plum tomatoes, halved
4 large thick slices of wholemeal
   bread
handful of rocket or assorted
   salad leaves
4 smoked mackerel fillets with
   peppercorns
sea salt and pepper

This is a light lunch or a quick snack. Smoked mackerel is available as plain fillets or covered in a crust of black peppercorns; choose whichever you prefer. This recipe is also very good with smoked trout or very lightly poached kippers.

1 Put the garlic into a food processor or blender with the pine nuts and parsley and blend to a rough purée. Add the lemon juice, olive oil and salt and pepper to taste and blend to make a salsa.

2 Put the halved tomatoes on a baking sheet and season lightly with salt and pepper. Cook under a preheated grill until the tomatoes are soft and lightly charred. Toast the slices of bread until golden brown and arrange on individual plates.

3 Cover the hot toast with the rocket and place a fillet of smoked mackerel on top so that the rocket wilts. Arrange the grilled tomatoes on top of the mackerel and spoon some of the green salsa over and around the fish. Serve immediately.

tuna teriyaki with pea & cucumber salsa

Preparation time: 15 minutes,
    plus marinating
Cooking time: 12 minutes
Serves 4

4 tuna steaks or mackerel fillets

Marinade:
4 tablespoons dry sherry
4 tablespoons soy sauce
2 tablespoons soft dark
    brown sugar
2 garlic cloves, crushed
1 tablespoon lemon juice
2 tablespoons sesame oil
pepper

Salsa:
250 g (8 oz) fresh peas
4 tablespoons virgin olive oil
1 garlic clove, crushed
1 tablespoon chopped mint
7.5 cm (3 inch) piece of cucumber
1½ tablespoons rice or white
    wine vinegar
salt and pepper

Oily fish are ideal for grilling since they do not dry out quickly with the heat. Tuna or mackerel are particularly good marinated in a teriyaki sauce and team well with this bright green salsa.

1 Make the marinade by mixing together the sherry, soy sauce, sugar, garlic, lemon juice and sesame oil. Add pepper to taste and whisk until well blended. Put the tuna or mackerel fillets into a shallow dish, pour the marinade over the fish, turn to coat well, cover and leave to marinate for 2 hours or overnight.

2 Make the salsa by cooking the peas in boiling water for 3 minutes. Drain well and refresh under running cold water. Put the peas into a food processor or blender with the olive oil, garlic and chopped mint and blend briefly to a very rough purée, or use a pestle and mortar.

3 Finely chop the cucumber and stir it into the pea purée with the vinegar, salt and pepper to taste.

4 Remove the fish from the marinade. Cook under a preheated grill for 5-6 minutes on one side then flip over and grill the second side for 2 minutes, brushing both sides of the fish with the marinade to stop them drying out.

5 Put any remaining marinade into a saucepan, bring to the boil and boil for 1 minute. Serve the hot tuna or mackerel on a bed of pea and cucumber salsa and pour a little of the teriyaki sauce over and around the fish. Serve with lightly grilled vegetables, such as fennel or courgettes.

salmon fish cakes
with spinach & poached egg

Salmon fish cakes are some of the finest and are quick to make and cook. If you particularly like raw salmon and have a very fresh piece of salmon fillet, you can make a very fine raw fish cake - a salmon tartare of very finely chopped fillet topped with tiny capers and finely chopped hard-boiled egg and parsley.

Preparation time: 20 minutes, plus chilling
Cooking time: 15 minutes
Serves 4

250 g (8 oz) King Edward potatoes, quartered
300 g (10 oz) salmon fillet, skinned and bones removed
1–2 tablespoons plain flour
6–8 tablespoons sunflower or groundnut oil
500 g (1 lb) spinach leaves
4 eggs
sea salt and pepper
lemon wedges, to serve

1 Put the potatoes into a saucepan of boiling water and boil until they are just cooked when pierced with a sharp knife. Drain well and leave to cool.

2 Either roughly chop the salmon or process it briefly in a food processor to make a coarse mince. Using a fork or the back of a wooden spoon, roughly mash the potatoes with salt and pepper. Add the minced salmon and mix together.

3 With floured hands, divide the mixture into 4 pieces and press firmly into 4 plump fish cakes. Coat each fish cake in flour and chill in the refrigerator for 1 hour.

4 Put the oil in a large frying pan and heat until hot. Add the fish cakes to the hot oil and cook for 3-4 minutes on each side.

5 Shake the washed spinach leaves dry, pack them into a saucepan and cover with a lid. Heat gently for 2-3 minutes or until the spinach has just begun to wilt. Drain the spinach thoroughly and season with a little salt and pepper.

6 Poach the eggs until just cooked. Remove the fish cakes from the oil and set them on individual plates, top each one with some of the spinach and finish with a hot poached egg. Serve with lemon wedges.

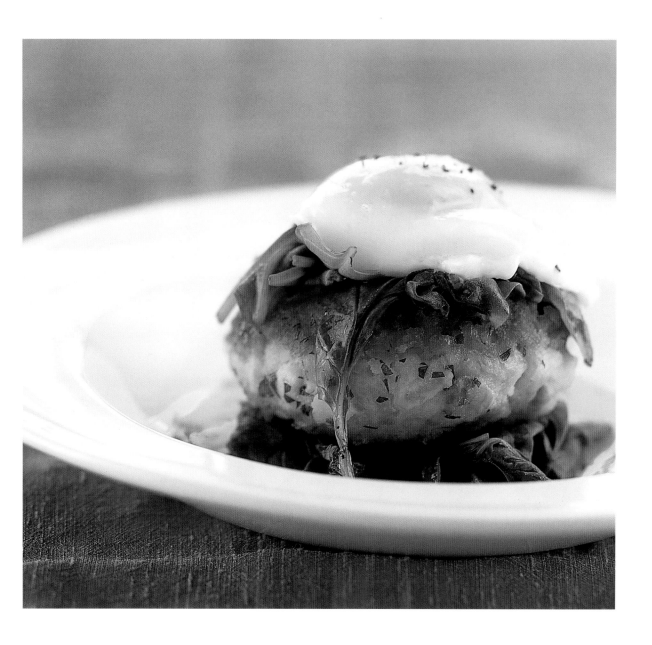

Fish oils improve the memory and other brain functions – so fish really is 'brain food'.

olive oil

This has been highly prized for thousands of years and in many different cultures both for its health-giving properties and its versatility in cooking. Its high levels of vitamin E make it a powerful weapon in the fight against disease and ageing.

Weight management

Paradoxically, olive oil can help fight the flab. It contains essential fatty acids which enable unwanted, stored fat to be removed from the system. However, it should still be used only in moderation if you want to lose weight, as excessive consumption will have the opposite effect.

Extended life span

There is increasing evidence that consumption of olive oil is linked to a longer and healthier life, as most cultures who use it regularly have a much better health record than those where animal fats are used instead. Its high and comparatively stable vitamin E content lowers the incidence of a number of the most common fatal diseases in the West, as well as their individual risk factors, reducing the risk of stroke, heart attacks, high cholesterol levels and arterial disease, and inhibiting the risk of blood clots and lowering blood pressure.

The high vitamin E content of olive oil is a potent antioxidant, fighting the free radicals that are a major contributing factor in the development of many diseases, including cancer. It also boosts the immune system generally, greatly enhancing its ability to ward off illness and infection. The fact that the vitamin E is consumed in the form of an oil means it is one of the easiest forms for the body to absorb and so few of its benefits are lost.

Vitamin E has a number of other important beneficial health effects. It improves the use of oxygen on a cellular level in the body and reduces unpleasant menopausal symptoms. It also prevents premature ageing, improving strength and stamina and keeping degenerative ailments, such as arthritis at bay.

A soothing oil

Olive oil is soothing and can calm inflammatory ailments. It is easily digested and encourages peristalsis (the muscular contractions of the bowel) and so is beneficial for a number of digestive problems. Wind, indigestion, heartburn and constipation are all eased by olive oil and it may also help heal ulcers. Some respiratory ailments, such as coughs and laryngitis, are similarly soothed.

A strengthening oil

The vitamin E in olive oil makes it important in strengthening key areas of the body. The muscles are one of the most visible of these and a lack of this essential vitamin will lead eventually to muscle wastage. Vitamin E helps to generate red blood cells and protects hormonal function and fertility. It also strengthens the collagen fibres in the skin.

Choosing, storing and using

Always buy pure, unprocessed oil. Choose cold-pressed oil – heating it during processing can reduce its vitamin E content. A dark glass bottle will help prevent oxidation. Keep the oil in a cool, dark cupboard and make sure it is tightly sealed.

Olive oil is stable at high temperatures, making it good for cooking. Use blended or virgin olive oil for cooking and extra virgin for drizzling and dressings.

The Benefits
- Boosts the immune system
- Combats free radicals
- Protects against heart disease
- Lowers blood pressure and cholesterol
- Protects fertility
- Keeps skin looking young

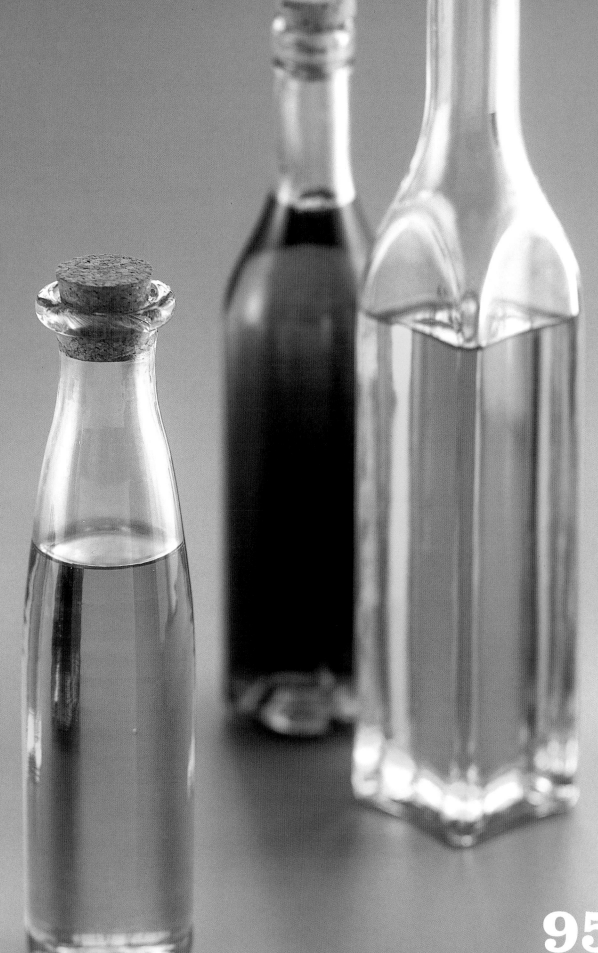

black tapenade with sea bass, flageolet beans & roasted tomatoes

Tapenade and pesto are the classic Mediterranean sauces - one from Provence and one from Genoa - that use olive oil.

Preparation time: 15 minutes
Cooking time: 20 minutes
Serves 4

125 g (4 oz) black olives, pitted
2 anchovy fillets
1 garlic clove, crushed
2 tablespoons capers
8 tablespoons virgin olive oil
1 teaspoon lemon juice
6 x 175 g (6 oz) thick steaks of
   sea bass, cod or other
   white fish
8 plum tomatoes
25 g (1 oz) basil leaves
6 tablespoons extra virgin
   olive oil
2 x 400 g (13 oz) cans organic
   flageolet beans, drained
sea salt and pepper
handful of basil leaves, to serve

1 Put the olives, anchovy fillets, crushed garlic and capers into a food processor or blender and blend to a rough purée. Add 5 tablespoons of the virgin olive oil, the lemon juice and salt and pepper and briefly blend once more.

2 Put the fish steaks into a roasting tin, arrange the tomatoes around them and drizzle with the remaining virgin olive oil. Roast in a preheated oven, 200°C (400°F), Gas Mark 6, for 10-15 minutes or until just cooked through.

3 Meanwhile, put the basil leaves in a saucepan with the extra virgin olive oil and heat very gently for 3-4 minutes or until the leaves begin to wilt.

4 Remove the pan from the heat, allow to cool, then blend to a coarse purée in a food processor or blender, or use a pestle or mortar. Add this basil oil to the drained flageolet beans, season with salt and pepper and set aside to allow the flavours to infuse.

5 Remove the fish from the oven and immediately spread each steak with some of the black olive tapenade. Serve the roasted fish on a bed of flageolet beans and topped with the roasted tomatoes and basil leaves.

olive oil marinated chicken with pumpkin mash & black beans

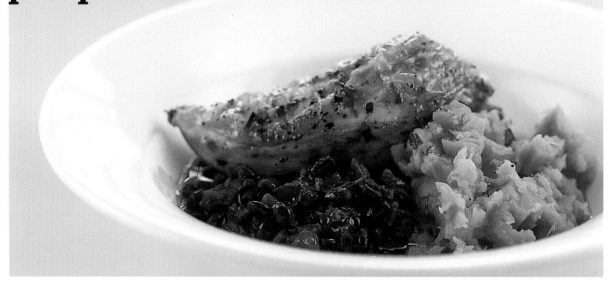

Preparation time: 20 minutes,
   plus marinating
Cooking time: 2 hours
Serves 4

150 ml (¼ pint) olive oil
6 garlic cloves, crushed
4 chicken breasts, on the bone
sea salt and pepper

Black bean and pumpkin mash:
4 rashers smoked bacon, diced
175 g (6 oz) black beans, soaked
3 garlic cloves, crushed
2 teaspoons thyme leaves
¼ teaspoon crushed chilli
475 g (15 oz) can organic tomatoes
2 tablespoons chopped coriander
4 tomatoes, finely chopped
500 g (1 lb) pumpkin
2 tablespoons virgin olive oil
250 g (8 oz) carrots
extra virgin olive oil, to serve
1 tablespoon chopped flat
   leaf parsley, to garnish

This is a rustic Italian meal of chicken slowly cooked in olive oil with braised black beans and a rough pumpkin mash.

1 Mix the olive oil with the crushed garlic, salt and pepper and pour over the chicken breasts. Coat well, cover the dish and marinate overnight in the refrigerator.

2 Fry the bacon in its own fat until crisp. Rinse the beans and put them in a saucepan with the garlic, bacon, thyme and chilli. Add the canned tomatoes and enough water to cover, bring to the boil and boil for 15 minutes. Cover and simmer for 2 hours, adding extra water if necessary. When the beans are tender, season with salt and pepper and add the chopped coriander and chopped tomatoes.

3 Transfer the chicken and marinade to a roasting tin, skin side up. Cook in a preheated oven, 190°C (375°F), Gas Mark 5, for 30-40 minutes, basting regularly.

4 Meanwhile, peel and deseed the pumpkin. Roughly chop the flesh and sauté in the oil for 2-3 minutes. Add the carrots and 8 tablespoons water, cover and simmer for 20-30 minutes until the pumpkin is reduced to a purée and the carrots are tender. Pour off any excess liquid and roughly mash the vegetables. Season to taste with salt and pepper.

5 Serve the chicken with the mashed pumpkin and black beans, drizzled with oil and sprinkled with parsley.

peppers

There are red, yellow, green and orange peppers and all of them have high levels of essential vitamins and minerals. They are powerful antioxidants and energizers.

ACE vitamins

Peppers contain very high levels of vitamin C, together with beta-carotene which is converted by the body into vitamin A (this is especially high in red peppers) and vitamin E – in fact, all the antioxidant vitamins are present in a single highly concentrated source. Peppers also contain zinc, one of the antioxidant minerals. This puts peppers high on the list of nutritious foods. They are especially protective of immune health. Because they are such a rich source of the antioxidants that fight off the degenerative powers of free radical cells, they protect against the risk of heart disease, stroke and many forms of cancer.

Energy and stress

Vitamin C is also needed for energy production, and including peppers in your diet will give you more energy. If you have a deficiency of vitamin C, it can show itself in a number of ways. The immune system becomes suppressed, making you more susceptible to colds and flu. It can often make you feel tired, but also prevent you sleeping properly. It can result in bleeding gums and mouth ulcers and can slow down the healing of cuts and wounds. Vitamin C cannot be stored in the body so it needs to be taken regularly to keep levels high. Smokers need extra vitamin C as cigarettes reduce levels of this vitamin.

Vitamin C will also help you deal with stress. Stress can come either from the tensions of everyday life and your emotional response to them or from the physical strain that is put on your body by a poor diet, a sedentary lifestyle and a host of other factors. Stress, as is well known, undermines the immune system, so the antioxidants in peppers will help to redress the balance. They help on another level too. The adrenal glands, which have to work overtime when you are under stress, need plenty of vitamin C to function properly and, of course, peppers have an abundance. They also contain magnesium, which is the most necessary mineral for the performance of the adrenal glands.

Stimulating good health

Peppers have a stimulating and invigorating effect on the system. They stimulate digestion, especially when eaten raw or as a juice, and prevent constipation. They also benefit the circulation. They improve the recovery rate from illness and also have a beneficial effect on the skin.

Choosing, storing and using

Peppers should have smooth, strongly coloured skin and be firm to the touch. Any with dried up or wrinkled skins are past their best. Buy organic ones whenever possible, store in the refrigerator and use within a day or two. Peppers can be eaten raw in salads or with dips, cooked in a wide variety of recipes or juiced. They make a surprisingly sweet and delicious juice, the red and yellow peppers being sweeter than the green. You can put the whole pepper into the juicer, including the seeds.

The Benefits
- Boost immune health
- Provide energy
- Help deal with stress
- Lower risk of heart disease, stroke and cancer

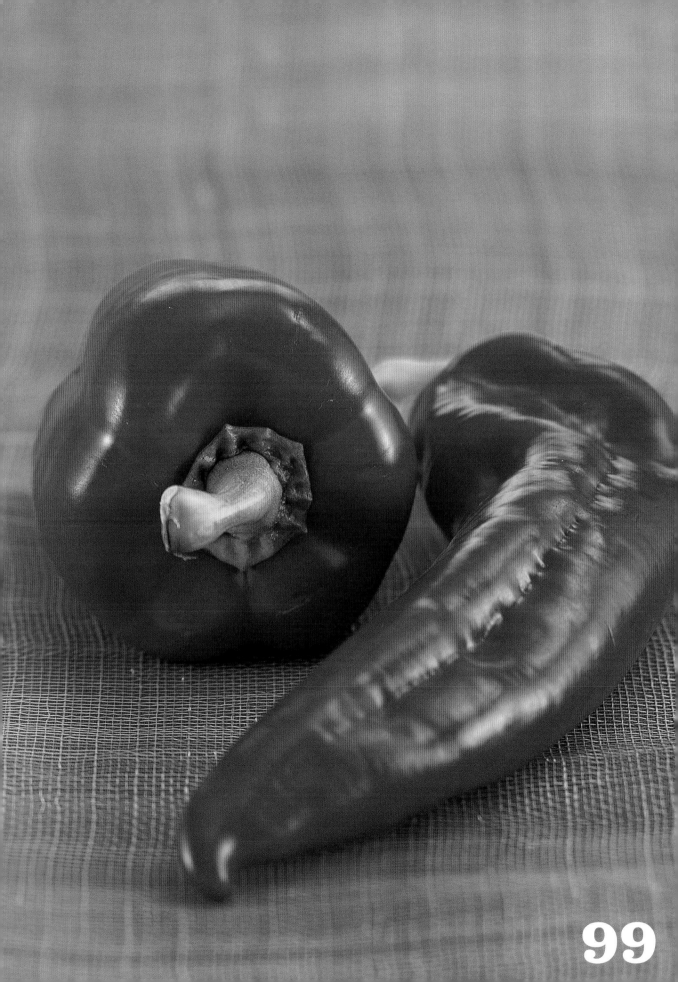

mixed combo juice

Preparation time: 5 minutes
Serves 2

2 red peppers
1 orange or yellow pepper
1 orange
2 celery sticks
25 g (1 oz) fresh root ginger,
    peeled and grated

Any vegetables or fruits, from beetroot, cucumber and apple to carrot, ginger and mango, can be blended together to make a wonderfully refreshing and highly nutritious raw juice. If you have a juicer, the juice will be smooth and thin, but if you use a food processor or blender the juice will be thick, since it contains all the fibre from the fruits and vegetables.

1 Remove the cores and deseed the peppers. Roughly chop the flesh and put it into a food processor or blender.

2 Remove the rind and pith from the orange. Cut the fruit in half, remove the pips and roughly chop the flesh, discarding any large pieces of membrane. Roughly chop the celery, then put the orange and celery into the food processor with the grated ginger and blend for 1 minute.

3 Add 200 ml (7 fl oz) water and blend for 1-2 minutes or until the juice is as smooth as possible. If you prefer a smoother juice, work it through a sieve. Serve immediately.

roasted peppers with millet & basil

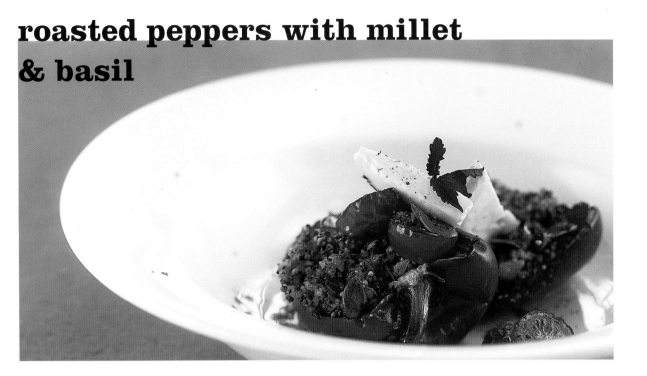

Preparation time: 15 minutes
Cooking time: 2 hours 10 minutes
Serves 4–6

3 large red peppers
175 g (6 oz) raw millet
5 tablespoons olive oil
1 onion, finely chopped
1 tablespoon chopped parsley
1 tablespoon harissa paste or
 pesto (optional)
1 tablespoon pumpkin
 seeds, toasted
15 g (½ oz) basil leaves
12 cherry tomatoes
sea salt and pepper

To serve:
thick slices of goats' cheese
basil leaves
extra virgin olive oil

Peppers are excellent roasted in the oven, which brings out their sweetness. Here they are stuffed with millet and cooked slowly. Serve with a salad or with a selection of dishes like a Greek mezze.

1 Cut each red pepper in half and remove the seeds and white membrane. Pack the pepper halves tightly into a roasting tin with the skin side down, like little cups.

2 Heat a frying pan until hot, add the millet grains and toast for 2-3 minutes, shaking the pan frequently.

3 In a separate saucepan, heat 2 tablespoons of the oil and lightly fry the onion until golden brown. Add the toasted millet grains, parsley, salt, pepper and harissa or pesto, if using. Add 450 ml (¾ pint) water, bring to the boil and boil for 5 minutes. Cover the pan and cook for a further 30 minutes or until the millet grains are soft. Add more water if they begin to dry out.

4 Stir the toasted pumpkin seeds and basil into the millet, then spoon the millet into the pepper cups. Cut the cherry tomatoes in half, put two halves on top of each pepper and drizzle with the remaining olive oil.

5 Pour 150 ml (¼ pint) cold water over the bottom of the roasting tin, cover tightly with foil and cook in the centre of a preheated oven, 190°C (375°F), Gas Mark 5, for 1½ hours.

6 Top the hot peppers with goats' cheese, basil leaves and drizzle olive oil over and around them.

seaweed & sea vegetables

Seaweeds and sea vegetables are some of the best available sources of a whole range of important minerals, including calcium, iron, potassium, copper, zinc, silicon and iodine.

Mineral treasures from the deep

Most edible seaweed grows in coastal waters where most forms of life contain iodine. This mineral is one of the reasons that sea fish and shellfish are so nutritious but, interestingly, seaweed contains even higher levels of iodine than fish. Iodine is needed for the thyroid gland to function properly; without it, the body's metabolism slows down, becoming prone to goitre. In the foetus, babies and young children, lack of iodine can also bring about developmental problems in the brain.

Sea vegetables have some of the highest levels of other important minerals too. Their high iron content helps in the formation of red blood cells. Potassium helps to keep blood pressure under control and supports the kidneys and the nervous system. Zinc is a powerful antioxidant mineral, vital for cellular growth and health and of great benefit to the liver and the to efficient functioning of the body's immune system. Magnesium is essential for healthy muscle and nerve functioning. The only problem mineral that seaweed often contains is sodium, but rinsing under running water for a minute or two should get rid of the salt.

Besides its mineral wealth, seaweed is also a valuable source of protein, particularly for strict vegetarians who do not eat fish. Seaweed is an effective detoxifier and is particularly valuable for removing dangerous heavy metals from the body. It also generally supports the heart and the nervous system. In addition, there is increasing evidence that including seaweed in the diet reduces the risk of developing cancer.

Choosing, storing and using

You can buy seaweed and sea vegetables from health food shops and, increasingly, from supermarkets. Usually it comes in a dried form which keeps indefinitely, though you can get fresh dulse which should be eaten within a day or two. Some seaweed comes covered in salt and should be rinsed thoroughly before use. Most dried seaweeds will need a brief preliminary soaking of about 5 minutes unless they are being included in a stew or soup. In all cases, only a little seaweed should be used as a flavouring for other foods. Seaweed and sea vegetables include the following:

Arame is usually available in a shredded form and can be steamed, sautéed or eaten cold. It is used in Japanese miso soup.

Dulse has a strong, salty taste and can be eaten raw if fresh, or if dried, soaked then cooked.

Kombu, a type of kelp, can be eaten raw or cooked and makes a good stock.

Nori, a processed form of laver, is usually toasted and wrapped around small rice balls in Japanese cuisine. It should be soaked before use.

Wakame should be soaked and then the central vein removed. It can be cooked in soups and stews or eaten raw in salads.

The Benefits
- **Detoxify**
- **Support thyroid function**
- **Support immune system**
- **Support heart function**
- **Support nervous system**

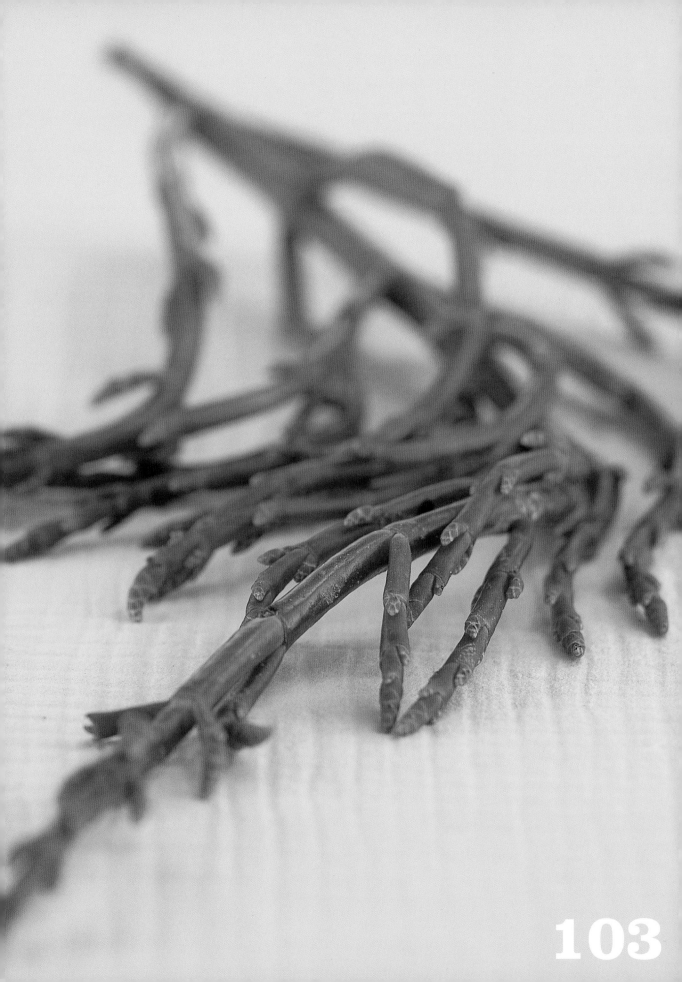

stir-fried arame seaweed with tofu

Preparation time: 10 minutes,
 plus soaking
Cooking time: 20 minutes
Serves 4

500 g (1 lb) firm tofu
25–50 g (1–2 oz) rice flour or
 plain flour, for dusting
10–12 tablespoons groundnut oil,
 for frying
15 g (½ oz) arame seaweed
2 garlic cloves, crushed
3 tablespoons light soy sauce
6 tablespoons mirin
2 teaspoons clear honey
4 teaspoons sesame oil
2 spring onions or 6 mangetout,
 finely shredded
boiled brown rice, to serve

Arame seaweed has a firm texture, which contrasts well with tofu. This is a simple stir-fry which can be assembled at the last minute once the tofu has been fried and the seaweed soaked. Serve hot with freshly boiled brown rice or leave to cool and serve as a chilled salad with grilled mackerel or teriyaki salmon.

1 Cut the tofu into thick slices and dust them in rice flour or plain flour. Heat 8-10 tablespoons of the groundnut oil in a frying pan and fry the pieces of tofu, two at a time, for about 2-4 minutes, turning them once or until golden brown on all sides. Remove the tofu from the oil and drain on kitchen paper. Reserve the oil.

2 Soak the arame seaweed in boiling water for 30 minutes. Remove the seaweed and reserve the soaking water. Roughly chop any large strands of seaweed. Strain the soaking water and put 6 tablespoons into a saucepan with the garlic, soy sauce, mirin and honey and heat gently for 5 minutes.

3 Heat the remaining 2 tablespoons of groundnut oil in a wok or large frying pan. Return the tofu to the oil with the seaweed and stir-fry for 1 minute. Add the mirin and soy mixture to the hot pan and stir-fry quickly. Add the sesame oil and shredded spring onions or mangetout and serve with boiled brown rice.

seaweed & cucumber salad with rice wine vinegar dressing

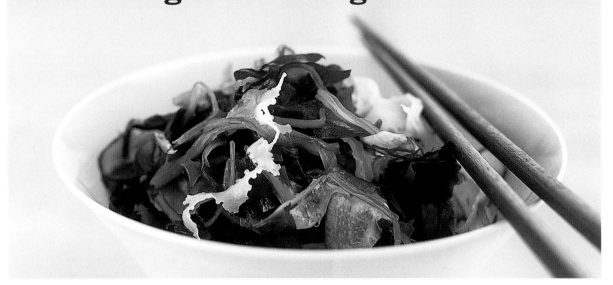

Preparation time: 10 minutes, plus soaking
Cooking time: 3–4 minutes
Serves 4

25 g (1 oz) mixed dried seaweed, such as dulse and sea lettuce
1 small cucumber
75 ml (3 fl oz) mirin
75 ml (3 fl oz) rice wine vinegar
2 tablespoons golden caster sugar
2 tablespoons lemon juice

Seaweed is packed with iron, calcium and potassium. This salad is best made with the mixed bags of seaweed and sea lettuces available in Chinese and oriental stores. Serve the salad as a starter or snack with miso soup or as a side dish with grilled fish.

1 Place the seaweed in a bowl, cover with cold water and leave to stand for 15-20 minutes to soften.

2 Cut the cucumber in half lengthways, then slice it very thinly into half moons. Drain the seaweed and roughly chop any large pieces. Put the chopped seaweed in a bowl with the sliced cucumber.

3 Mix the mirin with the rice wine vinegar and sugar and heat very gently in a small saucepan until the sugar has dissolved. Remove from the heat and allow to cool, then add the lemon juice.

4 Pour the dressing over the seaweed and cucumber and toss lightly. Serve in small mounds on individual plates.

seeds

Sesame, sunflower and pumpkin seeds are valuable sources of protein and essential fatty acids. Other beneficial seeds include linseed (or flaxseed) and psyllium seed, both superb intestinal cleansers.

Essential fatty acids

Sesame, pumpkin and sunflower seeds are rich sources of the essential Omega-3 fatty acids, while sesame and sunflower seeds also contain the Omega-6 fatty acids. Both of these groups of fatty acids must be provided by your diet, as your body cannot manufacture them itself and they are vital to your health. They are necessary for the regeneration of healthy cells and protect against blood clotting and the risk of heart disease. Essential fatty acids also nourish the skin, improve the symptoms of rheumatoid arthritis and may give protection against certain forms of cancer.

Cleansing and strengthening

All these seeds are packed with a wealth of vitamins and minerals. Sunflower seeds contain vitamins A, B, D, E and K, as well as the minerals calcium, iron and zinc. Vitamin E works with the essential fatty acids to give extra protection against the risk of heart attack, angina and arterial disease. Sunflower seeds are also thought to strengthen the eyesight and reduce the risk of cataracts. They detoxify the body generally and, in particular, remove heavy metals from the system.

Pumpkin seeds contain the B vitamins, calcium, iron, magnesium and zinc. Their high zinc content helps wound healing, while traditionally they are associated with prostate health and the prevention or reduction of bladder stones.

Sesame seeds contain high levels of vitamin E, folic acid, calcium, selenium, iron, magnesium and zinc. Their zinc content helps wound healing and growth and development. The zinc combined with high levels of selenium means sesame seeds are antioxidant and cleansing. They are also believed to strengthen the heart and the immune and nervous systems.

The intestinal clean sweep

Both psyllium seeds and linseeds are powerful intestinal cleansers. They are both gently laxative, preventing constipation and bloating, and also detoxify the bowel, removing parasites and bacterial or fungal infections. However, they are not harsh on the bowel and actually encourage the friendly intestinal flora. Linseed may also reduce certain menopausal symptoms, such as hot flushes, and lower the risk of breast cancer.

Choosing, storing and using

Buy seeds whole, rather than crushed, store them in an airtight container in a cool place and use within a few weeks. Seeds can be eaten in their raw state, though to bring out their flavour even more, toast them under a low grill or cook over a low heat in a dry frying pan, turning them over regularly so they don't burn. Both methods take only a few minutes.

Seeds are delicious as a snack, especially when mixed with dried fruit, or sprinkled into salads, soups and various other dishes. They can also be mixed with garlic and herbs to make dips. Tahini paste is an excellent creamy dip made from sesame seeds. Seeds are also used in baking and make excellent oils.

The Benefits

- Reduce risk of heart disease
- Help build healthy cells
- Protect against risk of cancer
- Improve prostate health
- Promote wound healing and growth
- Strengthen immune and nervous systems
- Cleanse digestive system
- Prevent constipation

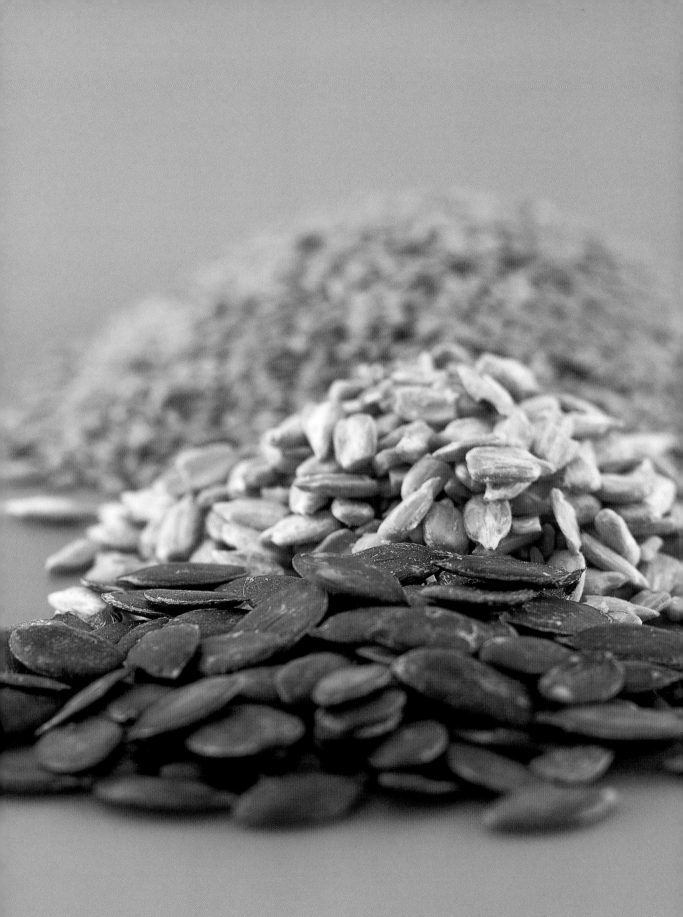

mighty muesli

Preparation time: 5 minutes,
    plus cooling
Cooking time: 20 minutes
Serves 6

50 g (2 oz) sunflower seeds
50 g (2 oz) pumpkin seeds
1 tablespoon sesame seeds
1 tablespoon desiccated coconut
2 tablespoons linseeds
75 g (3 oz) sultanas
175 g (6 oz) rolled oats
2 tablespoons soft light brown
    sugar

To serve:
assorted peeled and sliced fruit,
    such as papayas, mangoes,
    bananas or peaches,
    strawberries and apples
thick Greek yogurt

Packed with seeds, nuts and dried fruit, this first meal of the day will provide a nourishing start. Serve with yogurt and fresh fruit, or with milk or apple juice. To make in advance, increase the quantities and keep in an airtight container for up to 1 week.

1 Put the sunflower, pumpkin and sesame seeds on a baking sheet with the desiccated coconut and mix together. Roast in a preheated oven, 200°C, (400°F), Gas Mark 6, for 5-8 minutes or until beginning to brown. Remove from the oven and put into a bowl with the linseeds and sultanas.

2 Mix the rolled oats with the soft light brown sugar and spread over a baking sheet. Cook the oats in the oven for 10-15 minutes or until they begin to brown and stick together in clumps. Stir the oats occasionally.

3 Remove the oats from the oven and leave to cool for 5 minutes, then stir them to separate the clumps. Leave the oats to cool completely then add them to the seeds and sultanas. When completely cold, store in an airtight container.

4 Serve the muesli over thickly sliced papaya, mango and banana and add a large spoonful of yogurt.

mesclun summer salad with mixed seeds

Preparation time: 20 minutes
Cooking time: 3 minutes
Serves 4

250 g (8 oz) thin
    asparagus spears
2 ripe but firm avocados
2 tablespoons lemon juice
1 tablespoon sesame
    seeds, toasted
1½ teaspoons linseeds
assorted herb leaves – rocket,
    basil, flat leaf parsley, chervil
1 tablespoon pumpkin
    seeds, toasted
5 tablespoons olive oil
15 g (½ oz) basil leaves,
    finely chopped
sea salt and pepper

This is a bright green vegetable salad with a mesclun of herb leaves combined with avocado and asparagus spears and mixed toasted seeds. To retain all the vitamins and minerals make the salad and the dressing just as it is to be served.

1 Trim the asparagus spears, add them to a pan of boiling water and cook for 2–3 minutes. They will still be crunchy. Drain well and refresh in cold water.

2 Cut the avocados in half and remove the stones. Dice the flesh and add it immediately to the lemon juice, to prevent it from turning brown.

3 Remove the avocados from the lemon juice, reserving any juice, and add to a bowl with the asparagus. Add the toasted sesame seeds and linseeds and the rocket, basil, parsley and chervil leaves.

4 Put the pumpkin seeds into a coffee grinder or blender and grind until finely chopped. Mix the ground pumpkin seeds with the olive oil, any reserved lemon juice, the finely chopped basil, salt and pepper. Whizz in the blender or pound in a mortar. Drizzle the dressing over the salad and serve immediately.

Preparation time: 15 minutes
Cooking time: 12 minutes
Serves 4

4 x 150 g (5 oz) tuna steaks
1 tablespoon olive oil
4 tablespoons tahini paste
250 g (8 oz) soba
    (buckwheat) noodles
4 baby pak choi
6 tablespoons soy sauce
4 tablespoons rice wine vinegar
2 teaspoons clear honey
1 teaspoon sesame seeds, toasted
sea salt and pepper
lemon or lime wedges, to serve

Tahini paste can be found in large supermarkets, delis and wholefood shops. It is a ground sesame seed paste that can be spread on meat, fish or tofu. Keep the jar in the refrigerator once you have opened it since the oils in the tahini will turn rancid quite quickly if it is left in the light.

1 Season the tuna steaks with salt and coarsely ground pepper and coat with olive oil. Griddle or grill for 3-4 minutes on one side. Carefully turn the tuna steaks over and spread the top of each steak with some of the tahini paste. Griddle or grill for a further 3-4 minutes.

2 Bring a saucepan of water to the boil, add the soba noodles and baby pak choi and simmer for 5 minutes or until the noodles are just cooked.

3 Meanwhile, mix the soy sauce, rice wine vinegar and honey. Drain the noodles and pak choi and pour the soy mixture over them both and toss together. Put a mound of noodles on each plate and top with the tuna and pak choi. Sprinkle with the toasted sesame seeds and serve with lemon or lime wedges.

tahini on tuna with soba noodles & pak choi

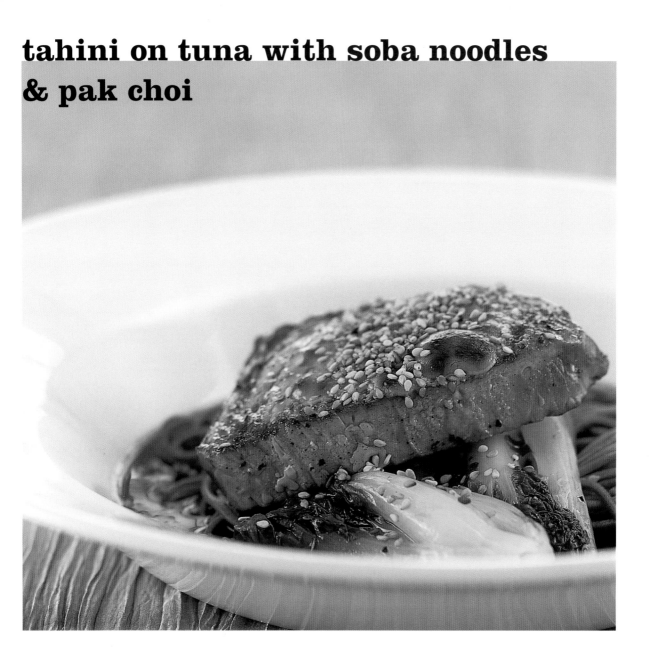

Seeds are packed with a wealth of vitamins and minerals as well as essential fatty acids which help to protect against the risk of heart attacks, angina and arterial disease.

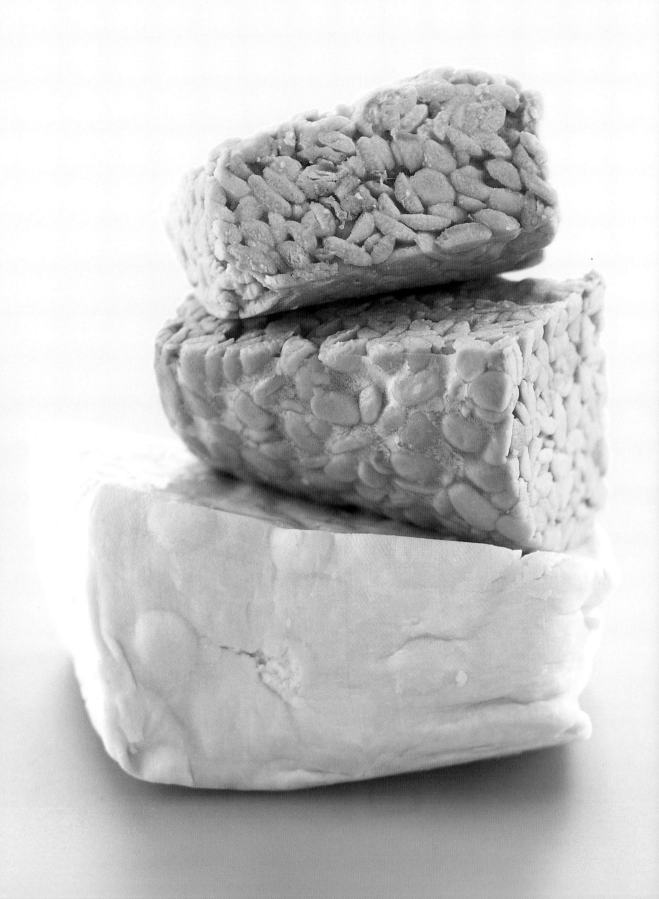

soya & tofu

Soya beans are the most nutritious of all beans, containing the essential Omega-3 fatty acids, the amino acids, phytoestrogens, protein, minerals and vitamins. They are available as beans for cooking, as a flour, a milk and as tofu.

Phytoestrogen protection

Soya is an excellent source of protein and, unlike many animal proteins, it reduces high blood pressure and cholesterol levels. However, it is now becoming best known for its cancer-fighting properties, as there is increasing evidence of its ability to protect against hormone-related cancers, including breast, cervical, ovarian, and prostate cancers. This is owing to soya's high content of phytoestrogens - chemicals, produced naturally in plants, that mimic the oestrogen hormone in women. An excessive level of oestrogen seems to be directly related to the risk of hormone-related cancers. Phytoestrogens diminish that risk.

Phytoestrogens are also extremely helpful for menopausal symptoms, such as hot flushes and headaches. Because phytoestrogens stabilize hormonal levels generally, they may also reduce both the physical and emotional symptoms of premenstrual syndrome (PMS).

Mineral benefits

Soya is an excellent source of many minerals, and tofu contains extra calcium too because it is made using calcium chloride - this may be why it is used traditionally in Japan for bone health in post-menopausal women. It has a high iron content, which contributes to healthy red blood cells; potassium, which maintains a healthy heart, kidneys and nervous system; magnesium, which regulates blood pressure; and phosphorus, which is essential for strong bones and teeth, a healthy heart and kidneys.

Soya fibre

Soya is rich in fibre and this encourages peristalsis, the muscular contractions of the bowel that prevent constipation or improve the problem if it already exists. Soya is a good source of the type of energy that is released slowly, safeguarding the blood sugar balance.

Choosing, storing and using

Buy soya beans that look plump and smooth skinned, preferably from a shop that has a high turnover. Store them in an airtight container in a cool, dark cupboard. Soak the beans in cold water, preferably overnight, but for at least 6 hours. Pour away the water, cover the beans in fresh water and boil for 2 hours.

Tofu is made from soya beans with the setting agent calcium chloride. It is available in three forms: silken tofu (the softest form, mostly used for dips and dressings), soft tofu (with a texture between the other two) and firm tofu (with the texture of hard cheese), the latter being the most commonly used.

Soya milk is now widely available and often recommended for people with a dairy allergy as a substitute for milk. Some soya milk has added sugar and this should be avoided. Soya cheese, a margarine-type spread, yogurt and cream are all available. Miso is made from the fermented soya bean and you can make stock or soup from it.

The Benefits
- **Reduce high blood pressure**
- **Lower cholesterol levels**
- **Protect against risk of hormone-related cancers**
- **Good source of non-animal protein**
- **Reduce symptoms of PMS and menopause**
- **Regularize blood sugar**
- **Lower risk of heart disease**
- **Prevent constipation**

tempe gado gado

Tempe is a fermented soya bean cake used mostly in Indonesian and Malay cooking, which is an excellent source of protein. It can be found in jars or in the freezer cabinets of oriental stores. If it proves too difficult to find, substitute firm tofu.

Preparation time: 20 minutes
Cooking time: 55 minutes
Serves 4–6

125 g (4 oz) waxy new potatoes
2 carrots
125 g (4 oz) bean sprouts
125 g (4 oz) green beans
175 g (6 oz) tempe
4 hard-boiled eggs
8 cherry tomatoes, halved
handful of coriander leaves

Peanut sauce:
125 g (4 oz) peanuts, roasted
1 small fresh red chilli
2 shallots, finely chopped
3 garlic cloves, crushed
3 tablespoons soy sauce
1 tablespoon lime juice
1 tablespoon groundnut oil
sea salt and pepper

1 First make the peanut sauce. Grind the peanuts in a food processor until they are quite fine, then add the red chilli, shallots, crushed garlic, soy sauce, lime juice and salt and pepper and blend for 1-2 minutes or until smooth.

2 Heat the oil in a saucepan, add the peanut paste and cook for 5 minutes, stirring constantly. Add 8 tablespoons water and stir well. Reduce the heat, cover the pan and simmer very gently for 30 minutes, adding more water if the sauce begins to dry out. Season with salt and pepper to taste.

3 Cook the potatoes in boiling water for 8-10 minutes or until tender. Roughly slice them and arrange on 4 plates. Scrub the carrots and cut into matchsticks, or grate roughly, then mix with the bean sprouts. Trim the beans, cover with boiling water and blanch for 1 minute. Drain well and refresh in cold water.

4 Heat a dry pan, add the tempe and toast on all sides until lightly brown. Remove the tempe from the pan and slice into cubes.

5 Arrange the drained green beans on the potatoes, then add the carrots and bean sprouts, hard-boiled eggs and cherry tomatoes. Drizzle the peanut sauce over the salad and top with the coriander leaves. Serve immediately.

fresh tomato & soya bolognese with egg pasta

Preparation time: 30 minutes
Cooking time: 50 minutes
Serves 4–6

1 kg (2 lb) ripe tomatoes or 2 x
    400 g (13 oz) cans organic
    tomatoes
2 tablespoons olive oil
1 onion, finely chopped
1 garlic clove, crushed
150 ml (¼ pint) red wine
1 tablespoon tomato purée
1 tablespoon tamari (thick
    Japanese soy sauce)
1 carrot, peeled
1 bay leaf
2 thyme sprigs
500 g (1 lb) soya mince or soya
    pieces, prepared according to
    packet instructions
2 tablespoons torn basil leaves
250 g (8 oz) egg tagliatelle or
    buckwheat noodles
sea salt and pepper

To serve:
basil leaves
Parmesan shavings

A fresh tomato sauce is an ideal base for GM-free, rehydrated soya pieces, cooked soya beans or pieces of fried firm tofu. Gently simmer together and serve with egg pasta or even buckwheat noodles.

1 Put the fresh tomatoes into a bowl and cover with boiling water. Set aside for 5 minutes then remove the skins and discard. Roughly chop the tomatoes.

2 Heat the oil in a large saucepan, add the onion and cook for 4-5 minutes until softened and golden brown. Add the garlic and cook for 1-2 minutes, but do not allow the garlic to burn.

3 Add the red wine to the pan, then add the chopped tomatoes or canned tomatoes, tomato purée, tamari, the whole carrot, bay leaf, thyme and pepper to taste and bring slowly to the boil. Stir well, then reduce the heat and leave to simmer for 25 minutes.

4 Add the soya mince to the tomato sauce with the torn basil leaves and simmer gently for 5-10 minutes. Remove the whole carrot and thyme stalks and discard. Season to taste with salt and pepper.

5 Bring a pan of water to the boil, add the tagliatelle or buckwheat noodles and simmer for 3-4 minutes or until al dente and just cooked. Drain well. Serve the bolognese sauce on top of the tagliatelle or noodles and topped with basil leaves and Parmesan shavings.

Packed with protein, this smoothie is good to drink at any time of the day as a quick snack. The linseeds can be replaced with spirulina powder.

Preparation time: 10 minutes
Serves 4

300 g (10 oz) tofu
2 bananas
125 g (4 oz) raspberries
**   (optional)**
1 litre (1¾ pints) white grape or
**   apple juice**
2 teaspoons linseeds

1 Roughly chop the tofu and put it into a food processor or blender. Roughly chop the bananas and put them into the food processor with the raspberries, if using, and half of the fruit juice. Blend until smooth.

2 Roughly grind the linseeds in a coffee grinder, or use a pestle and mortar, then add to the food processor or blender with the remaining fruit juice and blend until smooth. Serve immediately.

banana tofu smoothie

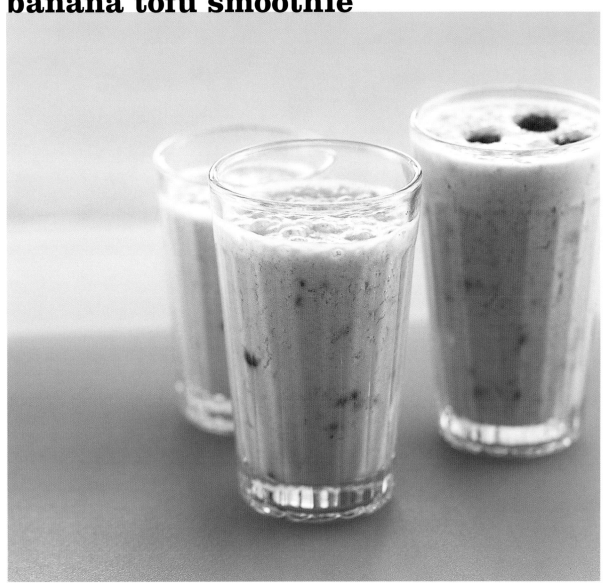

Soya beans are the most nutritious of all beans. An excellent source of protein, they will reduce high blood pressure and cholesterol levels.

spinach

One of the most nutritious of the green, leafy vegetables, spinach is beneficial for a wide range of ailments and protects and strengthens the body in numerous ways. It should not be eaten or drunk as a juice on a daily basis, however, as its cleansing effect can become too powerful. People with kidney or bladder stones should avoid it altogether because its oxalic acid content can exacerbate stones.

Immune health

Spinach is a powerful antioxidant containing high levels of beta-carotene, which metabolizes to vitamin A within the body, and vitamins C and E. It strengthens the immune system, making it easier to fight off infections, as well as neutralizing the toxins already present in our bodies from a variety of sources, such as pollution, stress, pesticides, cigarettes and over-the-counter drugs.

There is increasing evidence that the antioxidants present in spinach can also reduce the risk of both heart disease and stroke. Spinach may also lower the risk of certain cancers, in particular stomach and skin cancers.

A strengthening food

Spinach strengthens the body in a number of ways. It is high in calcium and improves the bones, teeth and gums. The chlorophyll that gives spinach its strong green colour also provides magnesium and vitamin K, which build healthy red blood cells. It contains folic acid, essential for protecting babies from the risk of spina bifida and for strengthening the nervous system, while its iron content strengthens the blood and prevents anaemia and its high potassium content regulates high blood pressure.

There may also be a link between spinach's potent antioxidants and sight, as people who eat this vegetable have a lower risk of both cataracts and age-related macular degeneration, which causes blindness. Spinach contains calcium, magnesium and manganese, all of which are believed to be beneficial to people with symptoms of osteoarthritis.

Spinach is a natural laxative, relieving symptoms of constipation, and also helps restore the potassium balance after diarrhoea. It is an energizing food, providing slow-release energy, and is effective in combating long-term fatigue.

Choosing, storing and using

Try to buy organic spinach whenever possible, and always look for a strong green colour and no sign of wilting. Keep fresh spinach in the refrigerator and eat within one day of purchase for the best nutritional value. Wash thoroughly and do not discard outer leaves as these are often the most nutritious. Cook spinach over a low heat in the water that remains on its leaves after washing – don't add any more to it. It will be ready in about 6 minutes. Spinach shrinks a tremendous amount when cooked, reducing to about one-tenth its raw volume, so you will need quite a large amount of it for most cooked dishes.

Young spinach is delicious raw in salads. Frozen spinach retains most of its nutrients. Spinach makes a powerfully cleansing and immune-protecting juice, but it is peppery and very bitter, so only a small quantity should be used, mixed with a sweeter juice, such as carrot or beetroot.

The Benefits
- **May lower risk of cancer**
- **Strengthens bones, teeth and gums**
- **Strengthens immune system**
- **Prevents and relieves anaemia**
- **Prevents and relieves constipation**
- **Normalizes high blood pressure**

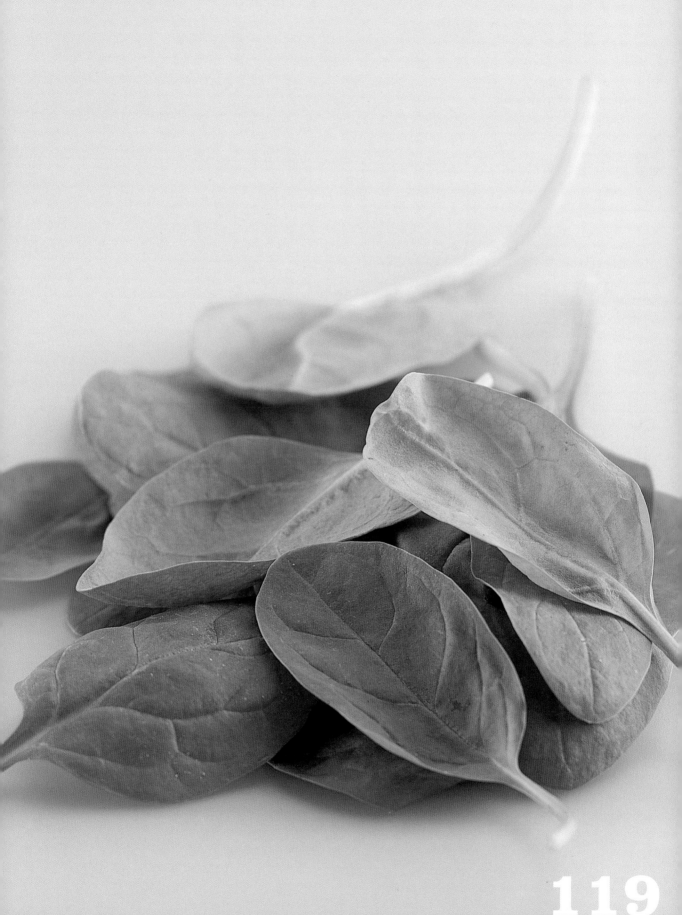

spinach with japanese sesame dressing

This is a very simple recipe that retains as much of the iron, vitamin C and beta-carotene in the spinach as possible. Served with a Japanese sesame dressing and boiled brown rice, it makes a light and delicious light meal.

Preparation time: 10 minutes
Cooking time: 1 minute
Serves 4–6

750 g (1½ lb) spinach, tough
   stalks removed and leaves
   thoroughly washed
6 tablespoons sesame seeds
1½ teaspoons golden
   caster sugar
3½ tablespoons light soy sauce
1 tablespoon mirin
2 tablespoons sesame
   seeds, toasted

To serve:
boiled brown or red rice
miso soup

1 Put the washed spinach into a large bowl or saucepan, pour boiling water over the leaves and blanch for 1 minute. Drain immediately and refresh under cold water to stop the cooking process. Drain well, then chop roughly.

2 Put the sesame seeds and caster sugar into a small food processor or blender and blend to a coarse purée, or use a pestle and mortar. Add the soy sauce, a little at a time, until it becomes a smooth paste. Add the mirin and blend well.

3 Pour the dressing over the spinach and toss well. Spoon the spinach into mounds in small serving bowls and top with the toasted sesame seeds. Serve with plain boiled brown or red rice and a bowl of miso soup.

spinach & saffron risotto

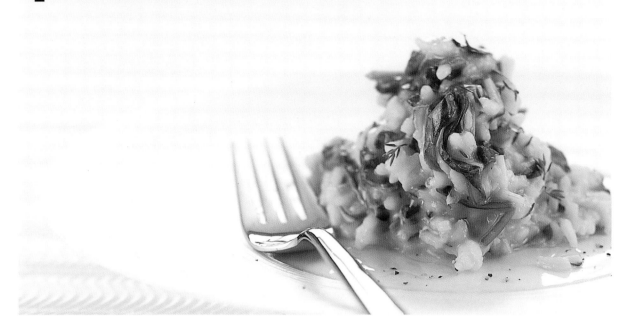

Preparation time: 10 minutes, plus soaking
Cooking time: 45 minutes
Serves 4

10–20 saffron threads
1 onion, finely chopped
3 tablespoons olive oil
2 garlic cloves, crushed
1 teaspoon thyme leaves
300 g (10 oz) arborio rice
1 litre (1¾ pints) boiling chicken
   or vegetable stock or water
375 g (12 oz) young spinach
   leaves, washed well
2 tablespoons extra virgin
   olive oil
50 g (2 oz) Parmesan cheese,
   finely grated
pepper

To serve:
Parmesan cheese shavings
extra virgin olive oil

Saffron and spinach risotto is a great Italian classic. In this recipe the spinach leaves are added right at the last minute, so they retain their green colour and as many nutrients as possible.

1 Put the saffron threads into a small bowl and cover with boiling water. Leave to stand for 30 minutes–2 hours to plump up and for the water to turn a bright golden yellow.

2 Put the onion into a large saucepan with the olive oil and fry gently for 8–10 minutes until golden brown. Add the crushed garlic and cook gently for 1–2 minutes, then add the thyme leaves, rice and pepper and stir them in.

3 Add half of the boiling stock to the rice with the saffron and soaking water and bring back to the boil. Cook for 20–25 minutes, stirring constantly, over a fast simmer. Add the remaining hot stock as the rice begins to dry out. Continue until all the stock has been used and the rice is soft and tender to the bite.

4 Roughly tear the spinach leaves, add to the hot risotto and stir together until the spinach leaves have wilted. Season the risotto with pepper to taste.

5 Remove the pan from the heat and add the extra virgin olive oil and the grated Parmesan cheese. Cover the pan with a lid and leave to stand for 5 minutes.

6 Stir the risotto once more and serve with Parmesan shavings and a drizzle of extra virgin olive oil.

tomatoes

The tomato is actually a fruit, rather than a vegetable, and one that figures prominently in the Mediterranean diet, which is renowned for its comparatively low incidence of heart disease. The tomato is used in many cuisines and is one of the most versatile of all cooking ingredients.

A hydrating food

Tomatoes have a particularly high water content – especially when eaten raw – and this helps to hydrate the digestive system and improve its function. Tomatoes are rich in salicylates, naturally occurring compounds that are associated with lowered risk of heart disease and help to prevent the blood from becoming too thick. However, salicylates may also increase the symptoms of hyperactivity in affected children so, if your child has this condition, it is worth eliminating tomatoes from his or her diet to see if this has any effect.

All-round antioxidants

Tomatoes contain all the antioxidant vitamins – A (beta-carotene), C and E – plus the antioxidant mineral zinc. This makes them an extremely powerful preventative food medicine, strengthening the immune system against infection and lowering the risk of cataracts, heart disease, stroke and various forms of cancer. Lycopene, an antioxidant flavonoid found in large quantities in cooked tomatoes, is thought to be particularly useful in the prevention of prostate cancer.

A fiery fruit

While they are widely recognized as a hydrating food, tomatoes can also overheat certain parts of the body in some people and herbalists therefore see them as a 'fiery' food. The people who most probably should avoid tomatoes are those who suffer from inflammatory conditions, such as osteoarthritis and rheumatoid arthritis, and in some case those with asthma and bronchitis. All these conditions can be aggravated by foods from the Solanaceae family, to which tomatoes belong, and which also includes potatoes, aubergines, courgettes, peppers and rhubarb. Paradoxically, tomatoes may help soothe inflammation of the liver.

Choosing, storing and using

Buy firm, red tomatoes when they are most nutritious and flavoursome. Choose organic ones whenever possible, or grow your own. Many varieties can be grown in pots, so you don't even need a garden. Freshly picked tomatoes are delicious in salads or as a juice. Store fresh tomatoes in the refrigerator and use within a day or two of purchase or picking.

You can buy canned, dried and puréed tomatoes too – all very useful for cooking and highly nutritious, though without the raw tomato's ability to rehydrate the body. You need to take a little care when buying tomato juice. Avoid canned juices as tomatoes are acidic and can leach undesirable metals from cans, glass bottles are much better. Check the ingredients label too. Tomato juice is often heavily seasoned with salt and this should be avoided. If you make your own tomato juice, you can achieve a pleasingly seasoned effect by juicing a couple of celery sticks at the same time.

The Benefits

- **Thin the blood**
- **Lower the risk of heart disease, cataracts and stroke**
- **Reduce the risk of cancer, particularly prostate cancer**
- **Improve the digestive function**
- **Strengthen the immune system**
- **Reduce liver inflammation**

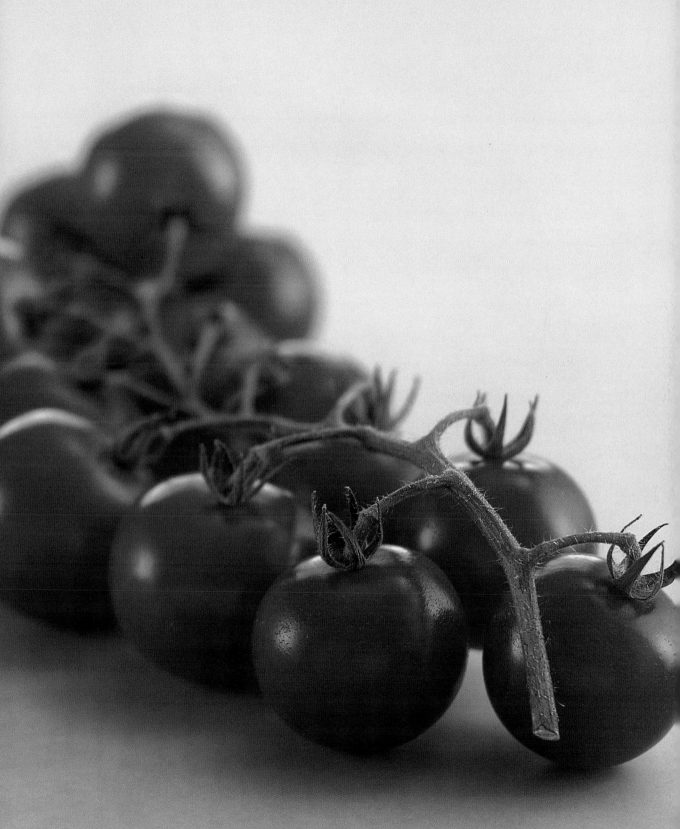

gazpacho with raw salsa

Preparation time: 15 minutes,
   plus chilling.
Serves 6

1 red pepper, cored, deseeded and
   roughly chopped
1 green pepper, cored, deseeded
   and roughly chopped
1.5 kg (3 lb) tomatoes, skinned
   and roughly chopped
2 garlic cloves, crushed
1 slice day-old bread,
   crusts removed
5 tablespoons olive oil
6 tablespoons white wine vinegar
1 teaspoon golden caster sugar
6–8 ice cubes, plus extra to serve

To serve:
1 red pepper, cored, deseeded and
   finely diced
1 green pepper, cored, deseeded
   and finely diced
1 small cucumber, finely diced
1 red onion, finely diced
flat leaf parsley leaves

This wonderfully cooling and refreshing soup made with sweet peppers and tomatoes is packed with flavour and vitality.

1 Put the red and green peppers, tomatoes and garlic into a food processor or blender and blend until a fairly smooth purée.

2 Roughly tear the bread into pieces and add to the tomato mixture with the olive oil, vinegar and caster sugar. Add 6 tablespoons of cold water and blend the soup until smooth. Add the ice cubes to the soup, then cover and chill in the refrigerator for 1 hour.

3 Serve the chilled soup with extra ice cubes and topped with the diced peppers, cucumber, red onion and parsley leaves.

tomato & apple pick-me-up

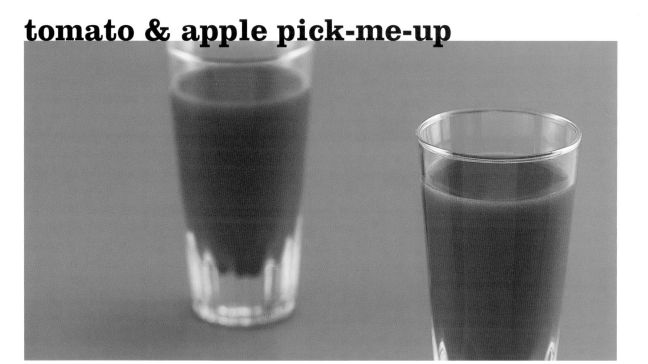

A simple and quenching juice for any time of the day. For the best results, it's well worth using organic ingredients.

Serves 1
Preparation time: 5 minutes

4 large tomatoes, roughly chopped
1 apple, cored and roughly chopped
1 celery stick, roughly chopped
4 basil leaves, finely chopped
1½ tablespoons lime juice

1 Put the tomatoes, apple, celery, chopped basil and lime juice into a juicer and whizz until smooth. Stir well.

2 Alternatively, put all the ingredients into a food processor or blender and blend well until puréed. If you prefer a smooth juice, strain the juice through a fine sieve into a glass.

3 Serve over ice for breakfast, at lunch time or as a virgin sundowner.

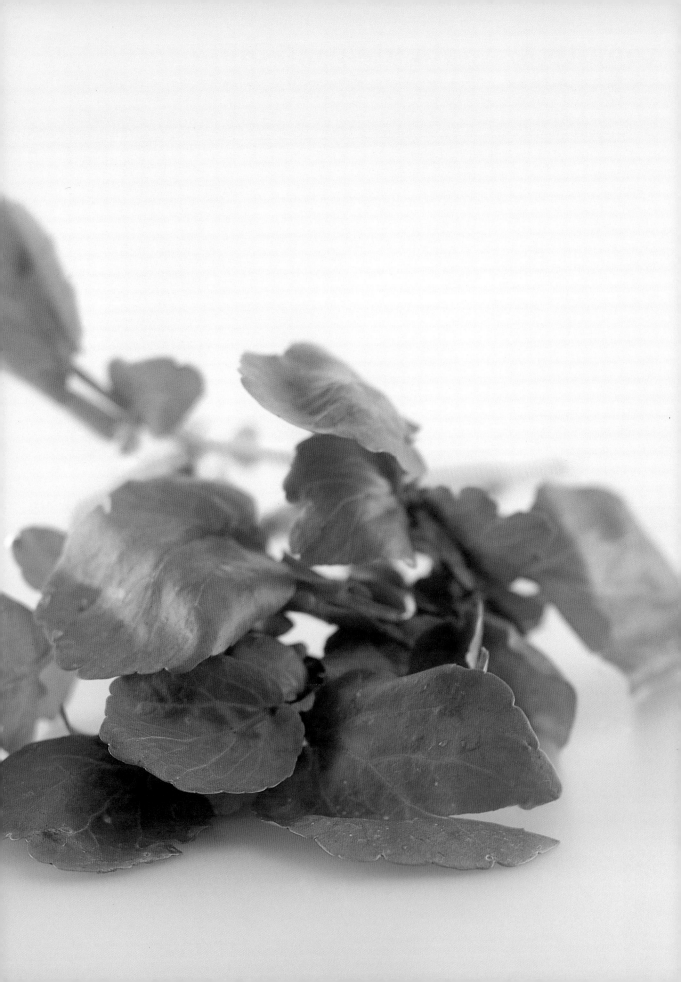

watercress

Watercress possesses potent health benefits, increased by the fact that is almost invariably eaten raw. It has very high levels of vitamins and minerals and is an excellent detoxifier and all-round immune builder.

Antioxidant power

Like spinach, with which it has much in common, watercress is a powerful detoxifier and contains all the antioxidant vitamins: beta-carotene (vitamin A) and vitamins C and E. Watercress, though, also contains the antioxidant mineral zinc, but it does not contain the oxalic acid that makes spinach unsuitable for anyone with kidney or bladder stones. In fact, watercress actually helps to dissolve such stones.

The antioxidants in watercress cleanse and fortify the immune system, increase resistance to a variety of ailments affecting the respiratory system – particularly colds, catarrh, sinusitis and throat infections – and reduce the risk of a number of the most common fatal Western diseases, including heart disease, stroke, various forms of cancer and cataracts. Watercress, which also contains iron, is renowned for cleansing and strengthening the blood, increasing the circulation and preventing or reducing anaemia. It is a natural antiseptic and antibiotic, and it regulates low blood pressure and lowers cholesterol levels. It increases energy and is a perfect food for people suffering from stress, who may feel fatigued as well as having a suppressed immune system.

The Benefits
- **Powerful detoxifier**
- **Boosts immune system**
- **Protects against risk of heart disease, stroke, some cancers**
- **Improves health of bones, teeth, muscles, heart, nervous system**
- **Boosts energy**
- **Improves skin problems and condition**
- **Dissolves kidney and bladder stones**

Green for beauty

Watercress is well known for its therapeutic effects on the skin. It combats inflammatory skin problems, such as eczema and psoriasis, and was used as a folk remedy for the removal of freckles and spots. It generally improves the condition of the skin. This may simply be part of a deeply cleansed system generally and show in a bloom of health in the skin.

As well as cleansing the blood and the immune system, watercress is also mildly diuretic and laxative, and stimulates liver, gall bladder, pancreas, kidney and bladder function. It acts as a tonic on the digestive system, improving appetite and the absorption of nutrients. It has a high iodine content, stimulating the thyroid function and supporting the growth hormones, and plenty of easily absorbed calcium for healthy bones, teeth, muscles, heart and nervous system.

It is rich in folic acid, which reduces the risk of spina bifida in unborn babies and strengthens the nervous system and blood cells of mother and child.

Choosing, storing and using

Look for, preferably organic, green leaves with no sign of wilting. Store watercress in the refrigerator and use it on the day of purchase, as it deteriorates quickly. Wash it thoroughly and use in salads.

You can also make a delicious soup from watercress, as well as a highly nutritious juice. In the case of juicing, though, you need use only a small amount – it yields a tiny amount of juice – because the flavour is so strong. Proportionally, it should make up no more than a sixth of the total of a mixed vegetable juice. The effects, though, are far reaching and it is one of the most healing and protective juices around.

wilted watercress
with garlic & nutmeg

Preparation time: 10 minutes
Cooking time: 5 minutes
Serves 4

3 tablespoons vegetable oil
1 garlic clove, crushed
750 g (1½ lb) watercress, washed
   and drained
1 tablespoon mirin
2 tablespoons tamari or
   soy sauce
¼ teaspoon coarsely ground
   black pepper
freshly grated nutmeg, to taste
15 g (½ oz) Thai or oriental basil
   leaves, torn

To serve:
cooked brown rice
soy sauce (optional)

This wilted watercress is good enough to be served on its own or it can be served as an accompaniment to other stir-fried dishes or oriental curries. To retain as much as possible of the vitamin C and beta-carotene, the watercress should be cooked only just long enough for the leaves to wilt.

1 Heat the oil in a large saucepan, add the crushed garlic and cook gently for 30-60 seconds until it is soft but not brown.

2 Add the watercress, mirin and tamari or soy sauce and stir-fry over a high heat for 1-2 minutes or until just wilted.

3 Season the watercress with the pepper and add grated nutmeg to taste. Add the torn basil leaves, then remove the pan from the heat. Serve with cooked brown rice and extra soy sauce, if liked.

watercress & pine nut salad with sweet mustard dressing

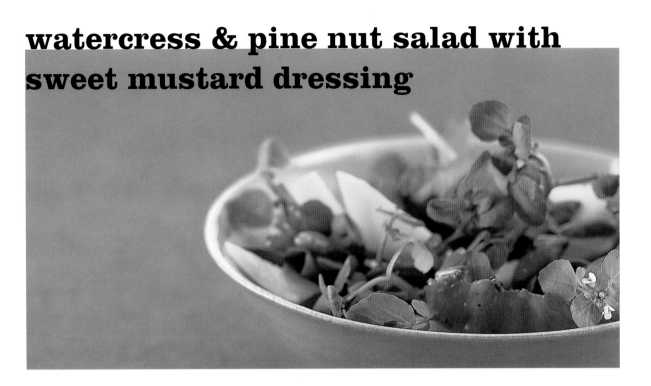

This refreshing, summery salad of fresh watercress leaves combined with sliced fresh mango and sweet pink grapefruit is packed with vitamin C and beta-carotene.

Preparation time: 15 minutes
Cooking time: 2 minutes
Serves 4

3 tablespoons olive oil
1 tablespoon white wine vinegar
1 teaspoon Dijon mustard
1 teaspoon soft light
　brown sugar
1 firm ripe mango
1 pink grapefruit
125 g (4 oz) watercress, washed
　and drained
75 g (3 oz) pine nuts or
　pumpkin seeds
sea salt and pepper

1 Mix together the olive oil, white wine vinegar, Dijon mustard, brown sugar and salt and pepper. Taste and adjust the seasoning.

2 Cut the mango into two either side of the central stone. Cut the mango flesh into dice or slices, then remove the skin. Remove the peel and pith from the grapefruit and slice the flesh into segments.

3 Squeeze the juice out of the grapefruit membrane and whisk 1 tablespoon of it into the dressing. Put the watercress into a bowl with the mango pieces and pink grapefruit.

4 Heat a dry frying pan until hot, add the pine nuts or pumpkin seeds and toast lightly, shaking the pan frequently. Remove the pine nuts or pumpkin seeds from the heat and scatter them over the salad with a spoon. Drizzle the dressing over the salad and serve immediately.

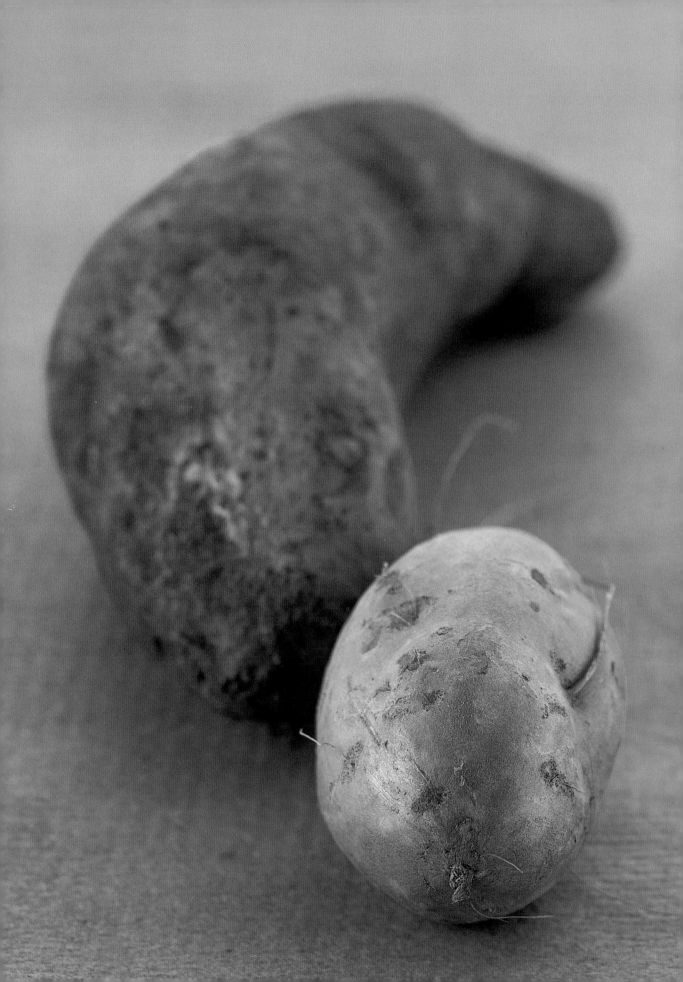

yams & sweet potatoes

These two dense root vegetables give a variety of health benefits, both being excellent detoxifiers, particularly of dangerous heavy metals. They both release carbohydrates slowly into the system, being energizing without producing the mood swings or food cravings associated with simple carbohydrates, such as white bread or pasta.

Yams

While sweet potatoes are in a number of ways the more nutritious of these two vegetables, yams have a particularly beneficial effect on female hormones. Because they stabilize oestrogen levels, yams can also regulate the mood swings as well as the numerous physical symptoms of both premenstrual syndrome (PMS) and the menopause.

Sweet potatoes

Sweet potatoes are full of antioxidants – beta-carotene (vitamin A) and vitamins C and E and the mineral zinc; the darker their orange colour, the more antioxidants they contain. These make sweet potatoes excellent detoxifiers and immune boosters. They cleanse the digestive system but also soothe it, so they are an ideal food to eat after digestive upsets of any kind. Their high antioxidant content makes them protective against the risk of cancer, heart disease and stroke. Sweet potatoes promote good circulation and are beneficial for ulcers.

They are the best low-fat source of vitamin E, which benefits cardiovascular health and also the skin, soothing inflammatory conditions such as eczema and psoriasis, and generally improving the complexion. There may also be a link between vitamin E and male fertility. Sweet potatoes also contain protein and a number of valuable minerals, including calcium, magnesium, potassium and phosphorus, which variously help to build strong bones, teeth and healthy blood cells, as well as supporting the nervous system, heart, kidneys and muscles and lowering high blood pressure. Their high iron content is beneficial for preventing and alleviating iron-deficiency anaemia. Sweet potatoes also have high levels of folic acid, which protects the unborn baby from spina bifida and strengthens the nervous system and blood cells of both the child and the mother.

Choosing, storing and using

Sweet potatoes and yams should be hard to the touch. Buy organic ones when possible and make sure the sweet potatoes are the variety with orange-coloured flesh. Store in the refrigerator and use within a few days. Scrub the skin of sweet potatoes and bake them whole. Yams have a very tough skin, almost like a bark, so you will need a sharp knife. Alternatively, you may find it is easier to bake them first and then peel them. After baking, sweet potatoes can be eaten just as they are, while yams are better mashed.

The Benefits
- Provide energy
- Prevent anaemia
- Promote digestion
- Improve immune health
- Reduce risk of heart disease, cancer, stroke
- Help to alleviate menopausal and premenstrual symptoms

131

sweet potato & coconut soup

This rich and filling soup is packed with vitamins and minerals. Instead of the homemade coconut milk, you can use 600 ml (1 pint) water and a 400 ml (14 fl oz) can of coconut milk, but, naturally, if you use fresh coconut milk it will be all the better.

Preparation time: 25 minutes, plus standing
Cooking time: 50 minutes
Serves 4–6

1 small coconut
4 tablespoons olive oil
2 onions, finely chopped
500 g (1 lb) sweet potatoes, peeled and roughly chopped
2 garlic cloves, crushed
7.5 cm (3 inch) piece of fresh root ginger, peeled and finely chopped
¼ teaspoon dried chilli flakes
sea salt and pepper

1 Using a corkscrew, drill holes in the three eyes at the top of the coconut. Pour the liquid out of the eyes and reserve. Crack open the coconut, prise out the flesh and grate it roughly.

2 Put the grated coconut into a bowl with 1 litre (1¾ pints) boiling water and leave to stand for 1 hour to cool. Squeeze and rub the grated coconut into the water, as if washing, to extract as much of the juice and oil from the coconut flesh as you can. Strain the liquid into a jug and reserve 2 tablespoons of the coconut pulp.

3 Heat the oil and gently fry the onion for about 10 minutes or until golden brown. Add the chopped sweet potato flesh and fry for 4-5 minutes or until the flesh has begun to brown.

4 Add the crushed garlic, chopped root ginger, dried chilli and the reserved coconut water and white coconut milk. Add the 2 tablespoons coconut pulp and salt and pepper and bring to a fast simmer, but do not boil. Cover the pan and simmer for 30-35 minutes.

5 When the sweet potato is tender, blend it, in batches, in a food processor or blender, then return to the pan. Check the seasoning once more then heat through thoroughly and serve.

gammon with yam mash & salsa rosa

Preparation time: 15 minutes
Cooking time: 45 minutes
Serves 4

750 g (1½ lb) yams
1 teaspoon cumin seeds
1 teaspoon coriander seeds
1 tablespoon sunflower oil
4–8 thick gammon steaks
3 tablespoons virgin olive oil
4 tablespoons thick plain yogurt
  or crème fraîche
handful of basil leaves
sea salt and pepper

Salsa rosa:
1 small red pepper
4 tablespoons olive oil
2 garlic cloves, crushed
8 olives, pitted and
  roughly chopped
15 g (½ oz) basil leaves
1 teaspoon Dijon mustard
2 tablespoons white
  wine vinegar

Yams are also a good detoxifier and anti-arthritic. They have a much drier texture than potatoes and take longer to cook, so add them to boiling water and keep it at a fast simmer.

1 Peel the yams and roughly chop them. Plunge them into boiling water and cook for 20-30 minutes or until they are soft when prodded with the tip of a knife.

2 Meanwhile, to make the salsa rosa, deseed and roughly chop the red pepper. Put it into a food processor or blender with the olive oil, garlic, chopped olives, basil leaves, mustard and white wine vinegar. Blend thoroughly.

3 Heat a dry pan and toast the cumin and coriander seeds until they release their aroma. Roughly crush the seeds in a mortar and reserve.

4 Heat the sunflower oil in the hot frying pan, add the gammon steaks and fry lightly for 3 minutes on each side or until cooked and golden brown.

5 Drain the yams well and roughly mash with the olive oil, toasted cumin and coriander seeds, yogurt or crème fraîche and salt and pepper. Serve the yam mash with the gammon steaks, topped with the salsa rosa and sprinkled with basil leaves.

yogurt

Yogurt is an excellent source of protein, a natural antibiotic and easily digested. It is particularly beneficial for intestinal health and the immune system. For maximum benefits, though, it is important to buy live yogurt.

Friendly bacteria

Yogurt is a living food. It is produced by the action of friendly bacteria on the sugars in milk (or lactose) that turns them into lactic acid. This is normally done by our own digestive juices and, as the lactose is often the cause of a food intolerance to dairy products, when milk becomes yogurt many people find it much easier to digest.

The Lactobacillus acidophilus bacteria in live yogurt are highly beneficial and needed for intestinal health. The intestines have their own bacteria, also known as flora, that are needed for proper digestive function, and live yogurt supports these. When intestinal flora levels fall, as they often do after a course of antibiotics, eating live yogurt regularly is the most effective way to restore the balance. Antibiotics can also cause problems, notably yeast infections, such as Candida albicans. Again, yogurt is of great benefit to Candida sufferers and should be eaten regularly.

Yogurt maintains intestinal health in other ways. It prevents diarrhoea, gastroenteritis and other bowel problems and it also helps the bowel recover more quickly if you have had diarrhoea or any other infection. It may also help to fight off the unfriendly bacteria that cause food poisoning and travellers' tummy bugs.

Immune protection

Yogurt is a very protective food and supports the immune system battle against bacterial infection on a number of levels. It protects against infections of the urinary tract, it helps prevent and aids in the healing of peptic ulcers and may even offer some protection against heart disease and reduce cholesterol levels. Its high calcium levels ensure strong bones and teeth and make it particularly beneficial for post-menopausal women who run the risk of losing bone density owing to osteoporosis. In folk medicine, it is associated with a long life.

Choosing, storing and using

All yogurt is rich in protein and calcium. Its other important health benefits, however, are provided only by live yogurt containing the Lactobacillus acidophilus culture. Many people who have an intolerance to milk are able to eat yogurt made from cow's milk because it is more easily digested owing to its healthy bacteria. However, there are also sheep and goats' yogurts available.

You can make your own yogurt easily or buy live, organic yogurt from the supermarket. Store yogurt in the refrigerator and eat it within a few days. Yogurt is extremely versatile. It is an excellent breakfast food and mixes well with fruit, seeds and cereals. It makes soups, stews and sauces thicker and creamier, but, as heating destroys its friendly bacteria, it should not be used during cooking but simply stirred in at the end.

The Benefits
- **Protects intestinal health**
- **Helps restore friendly bacteria after antibiotics**
- **Reduces vulnerability to, and speeds up recovery from, diarrhoea, gastroenteritis**
- **Reduces risk of osteoporosis**
- **Reduces risk of Candida**
- **Protects against bacterial infection**
- **Lowers cholesterol**

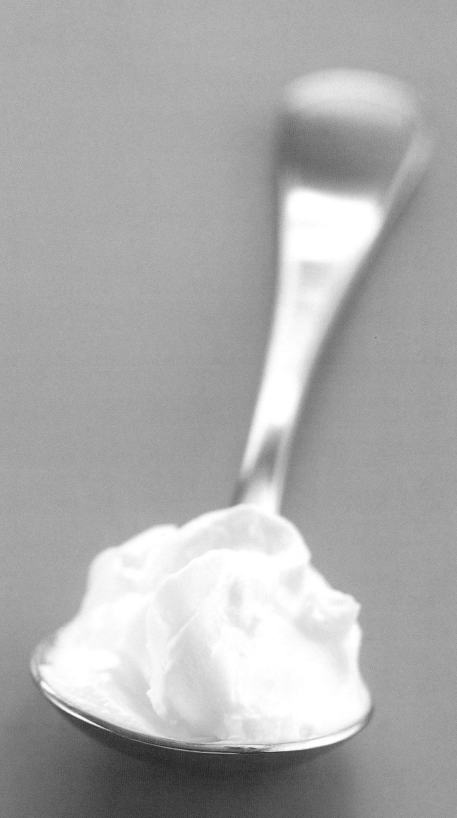

mango & cumin lassi

Lassi can be served plain or flavoured with a little salt, honey or sugar, or you can add any of the berry fruits, bananas or peaches to the basic yogurt mixture if you prefer.

Preparation time: 5 minutes
Cooking time: 2 minutes
Serves 4

½ teaspoon cumin seeds
1 small mango
300 ml (½ pint) thick
   natural yogurt
½ teaspoon clear honey
cracked ice, to serve

1 Heat a small frying pan, add the cumin seeds and toast until they release their aroma. Remove the pan from the heat and allow to cool.

2 Cut the mango into two either side of the stone. Slash the flesh in a criss-cross pattern. Remove the diced flesh from the skin and put it into a food processor or blender. Cut any remaining mango flesh from around the stone and add to the food processor. Blend with the cumin seeds to a smooth purée.

3 Add the yogurt and honey to the blender with 300 ml (½ pint) iced water and blend until smooth.

4 Pour the lassi over tall tumblers of cracked ice and serve immediately.

lemon & yogurt dressing with tandoori chicken kebabs

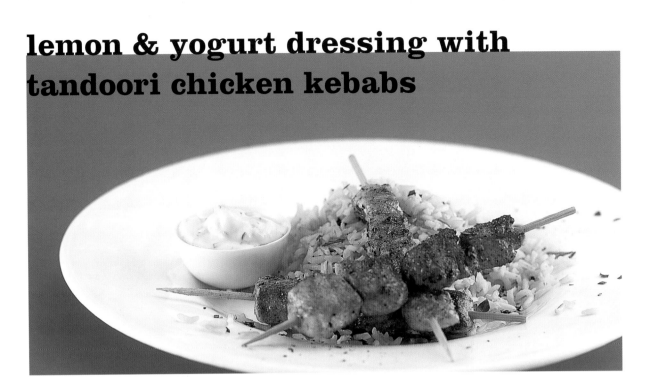

Preparation time: 15 minutes,
   plus marinating
Cooking time: 8 minutes
Serves 4

500 g (1 lb) chicken fillets
3 tablespoons groundnut or
   sunflower oil
3 garlic cloves, crushed
1 teaspoon ground cumin
1 teaspoon ground coriander
1 teaspoon hot paprika
½ teaspoon ground turmeric
150 ml (¼ pint) natural yogurt
3 tablespoons lemon juice
3 tablespoons grated cucumber,
   well drained
1 tablespoon chopped dill
½ teaspoon Dijon mustard
½ teaspoon clear honey
sea salt and pepper

To serve:
500 g (1 lb) cooked brown rice
handful of mixed salad leaves

This light and tangy lemon dressing laced with fresh dill and grated cucumber is a soothing addition to plainly grilled chicken kebabs. Make the kebabs in advance and leave them to marinate in the refrigerator overnight.

1 Cut the chicken into cubes or thin strips and weave on to thin kebab sticks (if you are using wooden sticks, first soak them in cold water for 30 minutes).

2 Mix the oil with the crushed garlic, cumin, coriander, paprika, turmeric and salt and pepper, and pour over the chicken. Coat the kebabs in the marinade, cover and chill in the refrigerator for 2 hours or overnight.

3 Combine the yogurt with the lemon juice, grated cucumber, chopped dill, Dijon mustard and honey. Mix well and season with salt and pepper.

4 Lift the chicken kebabs out of the marinade and cook under a preheated grill or on a griddle for 2–3 minutes on all sides (depending on the thickness of the chicken pieces). Check that the chicken is cooked right through.

5 Serve the kebabs on a bed of cooked brown rice and a handful of mixed salad leaves. Spoon the yogurt dressing over the kebabs and serve.

glossary

A, C and E vitamins The vitamins that are especially beneficial for their **antioxidant** effects.

Adrenal glands These are located above the kidneys and secrete adrenaline, a hormone that stimulates the heart in response to stress.

Allicin A substance found in garlic that dilates blood vessels and so reduces the risk of blood clots.

Allergy A sensitivity to specific substances, such as foods, pollen, pollution or drugs, causing such symptoms as rashes, breathing problems and congested sinuses. The reaction usually develops soon after exposure. In severe cases, allergic reactions can be fatal. See also **food intolerance**.

Amino acids The building blocks of **proteins**. There are twenty of them, twelve of which we can synthesize in our bodies. The other eight, the essential amino acids, have to be obtained from foods containing protein.

Anaemia Condition in which the haemoglobin in the blood is at reduced levels, lowering the blood's oxygen-carrying capacity. It is caused by various conditions, including lack of iron or vitamin B6, B12, C, folic acid, protein or copper in the diet, or excessive menstrual bleeding. The symptoms include pallor, weakness, depression and low resistance to infections.

Antibacterial Applies to substances that kill bacteria, but not viruses.

Antibiotics Substances that are capable of destroying or stopping the growth of bacteria and other microorganisms. There is increasing concern that the routine inclusion of antibiotics in animal feeds in order to increase yield may be leading to the occurrence of antibiotic-resistant bacteria (the so-called superbugs) and, when eaten by humans, lowers our own immune systems. Some may also kill friendly bacteria in the digestive tract.

Antibodies Proteins that work as part of the immune system. They are made by some white blood cells and target 'foreign' invaders or antigens, such as those belonging to viruses. After having been exposed once to a particular infection, the body 'remembers' the foreign protein and can react more quickly to it, fighting off the infection.

Antimicrobial Refers to substances that kill both bacteria and viruses.

Antioxidants Natural substances found in foods that help to prevent **oxidation** by mopping up **free radicals**. This leads to better general health and is thought to slow down the ageing processes in the body.

Antiseptic Refers to substances that prevent the growth or spread of microorganisms, inhibiting their action (without killing them).

Antiviral Applies to substances that kill viruses but not bacteria.

Arame A Japanese seaweed.

Beta-carotene An antioxidant found in many red and orange fruits. The body converts it to vitamin A.

Caffeine A mildly addictive substance found in coffee, tea, cocoa and cola drinks. It stimulates the central nervous system and heart, and is a **diuretic**. It increases alertness, but in excessive amounts can cause insomnia.

Calcium A vital constituent of human bones and teeth. It also performs an important role in sending nerve impulses to and from the brain, and in the contraction of muscles. Long-term deficiency may cause bone problems in later life, especially for post-menopausal women.

Carbohydrate (simple and complex) There are two types of carbohydrate foods: simple carbohydrates - **sugars** - and complex carbohydrates found in **starchy foods**, such as those found in potatoes and rice. In a balanced diet, about half of the body's energy intake should come in the form of complex carbohydrates.

Carcinogens Any cancer-triggering substance.

Chlorophyll The green pigment found in plants that conducts photosynthesis.

Cholesterol There are two types of cholesterol: High-density lipoprotein (HDL cholesterol), which is beneficial as it reduces blood cholesterol and Low-density lipoprotein (LDL cholesterol), which is dangerous as it encourages the deposit of cholesterol on the walls of blood vessels.

Copper A mineral that performs an important role in haemoglobin and bone formation.

Detoxification A process of removing toxins from the body.

Diuretics Chemicals that cause an increase in urine production by the kidneys, so dehydrating the body.

Dulse An edible seaweed from the Atlantic Ocean.

Enzymes Proteins involved in the chemical processes in the body, breaking down or synthesizing chemical compounds. Most exist within cells, except those in the digestive system.

Fats Some fat is necessary in the diet, and it is an important source of some vitamins. There are three main types of fats:
  • Saturated fats are found in animal foods and should be avoided if possible as they encourage the deposit of fatty plaque and bad LDL **cholesterol** on the walls of blood vessels.
  • Monounsaturated fats are good for frying as they can be heated to higher temperatures without degenerating. They are particularly good at maintaining correct levels of good HDL **cholesterol**.
  • Polyunsaturated fatty acids. See **Omega 3 alpha-linolenic fatty acid** and **Omega 6 lineoleic fatty acid**.

Fibre The indigestible parts of plant foods, which pass through the digestive system, absorbing water and accelerating elimination of waste.

Fibroids Growths of muscular tissue in the uterus. Although they are not cancerous, they can sometimes cause excessive menstrual bleeding, which may in turn lead to **anaemia**.

Folic acid Vitamin used in nucleic acid metabolism, lack in pregnancy can cause anaemia in the mother-to-be and spina bifida in the baby.

Food groups Five basic food types that combine to make up a healthy diet: fruit and vegetables; meat, fish and other protein sources; dairy foods; **starchy foods** and high-fat and sugary foods. See also **protein**, **fat** and **sugars**.

Food intolerance An adverse reaction to substances in food. The symptoms are not as immediate as those of an **allergy**, and include joint pains, rashes, stomach disorders and headaches.

Free radicals Abnormal, electro-chemically imbalanced molecules produced by the body as a natural waste product. They can set off a damaging chain reaction of **oxidization** within the body.

Free-radical scavengers Substances, such as **antioxidants**, that 'mop up' **free radicals**, and slow down their ability to increase.

Genetically modified food (GM food) Food that has had its DNA deliberately altered in a laboratory to improve it in some way, e.g., to increase disease resistance or improve yield.

High-density lipoproteins (HDL), see **Cholesterol**.

Hormones Chemical messengers produced in minute amounts in living organisms. Imbalances can cause such conditions as diabetes.

Hormone function The body's hormone system regulates all of its functions, using **hormones** as messengers.

Iodine Chemical important in thyroid function, which controls many of the body's **enzyme** systems. It is found in most plants, particularly seaweeds, as well as seafoods.

Iron A vital constituent of haemoglobin in the blood. Iron deficiency is one of the primary causes of **anaemia**. Mild deficiency causes problems in concentrating and a lowered resistance to infection.

Juicing The process of making fresh juice from raw fruit and vegetables in order to retain as many of the nutrients as possible.

Kombu A type of kelp seaweed.

Linoleic acid, see **Omega 6 linoleic fatty acid**.

Low-density lipoproteins (LDL), see **Cholesterol**.

Magnesium Necessary for bone growth and maintenance, as well as for obtaining energy from food. The effects of magnesium deficiency include depression, exhaustion, weakened muscles and heart problems.

Manganese A mineral that helps the body to utilize energy from food and aids **antioxidants**.

Nori A processed form of laver seaweed.

Nutrients The vital substances that cannot be synthesized by the body. See **Food groups**.

Nutrition The process of absorbing and processing the vital **nutrients** from food.

Omega 3 essential fatty acid (alpha-linolenic fatty acid) This fatty acid may help to reduce the risk of heart attacks. It is found in such sources as oily fish.

Omega 6 linoleic fatty acid (Linoleic acid) This fatty acid is thought to reduce blood cholesterol levels. It is found in nuts and seeds.

Organic foods Organic fruit and vegetables that have been grown without the use of synthetic pesticides, fertilizers or fungicides. Organic meat comes from animals raised without routine antibiotics or growth hormones.

Oxalic acid A poisonous substance found in many foods, such as spinach. It can aggravate kidney or bladder stones, so people with these conditions should avoid foods containing it.

Oxidization A process that occurs naturally within the body. **Free radicals** take a hydrogen ion from nearby molecules, which then do the same giving rise to a chain reaction within the body, that can lead to tissue damage. This chain reaction can be stopped by eating foods that are rich in **free-radical scavengers** that have an **antioxidant** effect.

Papain An enzyme found in papayas, which helps in digesting protein.

Pectin A soluble fibre that occurs in many ripe fruits and vegetables. It helps in maintaining bowel function.

Phosphorus Works along with **calcium** to maintain strong bones and teeth. It is also necessary for the body to process B vitamins and to obtain energy from food.

Phytoestrogens Substances found in plants which are similar to animal oestrogens. They are thought to help reduce some of the symptoms of pre-menstrual syndrome and the menopause.

Potassium Regulates the fluid levels in the body, so important in governing blood pressure. It cannot be stored in the body and so must be obtained regularly. Deficiency causes weakness, confusion and thirst. Severe lack causes high blood pressure.

Protein Used in the structure, repair and maintenance of cells. Essential for growth. All of the essential **amino acids** are found in meat, fish and dairy products, but only some of them in plant sources.

Salt Although salt (sodium chloride) is vital to health, the western diet almost invariably contains too much of it because it is used as a preservative in many processed foods.

Selenium Vital to the immune system, working together with **vitamin E**. Lack of it may also result in reduced fertility in men.

Silicon Plays a role in the formation of bone, cartilage and arterial walls. Deficiency may be a factor in cardiovascular disease.

Starchy foods The best source of carbohydrates in the diet. About half of the body's daily energy intake should come from starchy foods such as brown rice and potatoes.

Sugar Simple carbohydrates with little nutritional value. Some are found in fruits and vegetables, but the western diet contains too many refined sugars in sweets and drinks and in processed foods where it is used as a preservative.

Sulphuraphane A substance that is effective in removing carcinogens from the body. It is found in broccoli.

Systemic fungicides and pesticides These are chemicals that are absorbed throughout a plant, including its stems, leaves fruit or tubers. Simply washing the food before cooking or eating does not remove the chemicals.

Tannin A substance found in tea. It reduces the ability of the body to absorb iron.

Thyroid gland This gland secretes hormones that control growth and metabolism.

Toxins Harmful substances that may be taken in with food, or created by the body as a waste product.

Tryptophan One of the essential **amino acids**.

Vitamin A Important for eyesight, growth, skin and other tissues, such as the mucous membranes in the nose and lungs. Deficiency causes poor vision where there are low light levels, skin problems and susceptibility to infection.

Vitamin B1 (Thiamine) Used in processing carbohydrates and fats and for healthy nerves and muscles. Deficiency leads to problems in sleep, concentration, depression and irritability and in the long term nerve damage, muscle wastage and memory loss.

Vitamin B2 (Riboflavin) Vital for children's growth, repairing and maintaining tissues and obtaining energy from food. Symptoms of deficiency include skin problems and itchy eyes.

Vitamin B3 (Niacin) Used by the body in processing waste and in metabolizing fatty acids. Mild deficiency causes lack of energy and depression.

Vitamin B5 (Pantothenic acid) Used to process energy from fats and carbohydrates. Deficiency causes numbness in the feet, dizziness, tiredness, upset stomach, headaches and irritability.

Vitamin B6 (Pyridoxine) Used in processing and synthesizing proteins. Deficiency may cause depression, skin problems, irritability and nerve inflammation.

Vitamin B12 Vital for making DNA and RNA in every cell and in blood-cell formation. Mild deficiency causes anaemia.

Vitamin C (Ascorbic acid) Essential for healing wounds and general health. Symptoms of deficiency include poor general health, poor sleep patterns, aching joints and irritability.

Vitamin D Used in the process of obtaining calcium, so is important for bones, muscles and teeth. Deficiency in growing children leads to rickets and in adults to weak bones and muscle wastage.

Vitamin E Powerful antioxidant. Protects against heart attacks, strokes and some cancers.

Vitamin K Vital for the proteins that clot blood.

Vitamins Essential substances that the body has to obtain from food. Some (A, D, E and B12) can be stored in the body, but most of the B vitamins, C and K have to be eaten on a daily basis. See individual Vitamins.

Wakame A Japanese seaweed.

Zinc Vital for a healthy immune system, growth and tissue repair. Lack of it may result in skin problems, a depressed immune system, slow growth and loss of appetite.

index

acknowledgements

Picture credits
Octopus Publishing Group Ltd./Jeremy Hopley 1, 2-3, 7, 8, 9 top left, 9 bottom right, 10 left, 10 right, 11, 12, 13 left, 13 right, 14, 15, 16, 17, 18-19, 22-23, 25, 26-27, 29, 30-31, 33, 34-35, 37, 38-39, 43, 44-45, 47, 48-49, 51, 52-53, 55, 56-57, 61, 62-63, 65, 66-67, 71, 72-73, 77, 78-79, 83, 84-85, 87, 88-89, 93, 94-95, 97, 98-99, 101, 102-103, 105, 106-107, 111, 112-113, 117, 118-119, 121, 122-123, 125, 126-127, 129, 130-131, 133, 134-135, 137

Commissioning Editor: Nicola Hill
Copy-editor: Anne Crane
Production Controller: Jo Sim
Photographer: Jeremy Hopley
Stylist: Angela Swaffield
Home Economist: Oona van den Berg